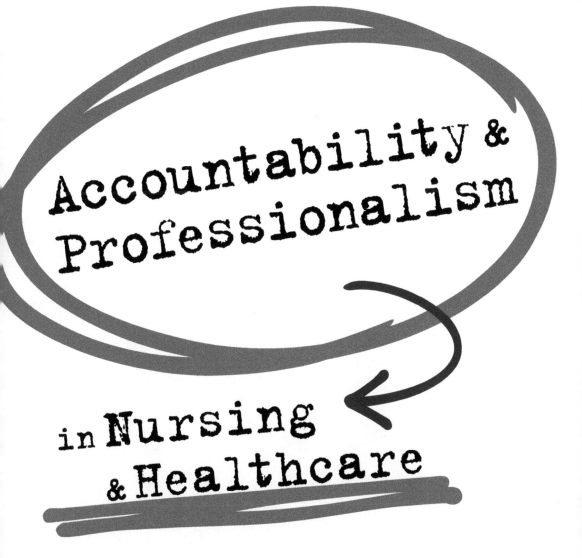

Accountability & Professionalism

in Nursing & Healthcare

Sara Miller McCune founded SAGE Publishing in 1965 to support the dissemination of usable knowledge and educate a global community. SAGE publishes more than 1,000 journals and over 800 new books each year, spanning a wide range of subject areas. Our growing selection of library products includes archives, data, case studies and video. SAGE remains majority owned by our founder and after her lifetime will become owned by a charitable trust that secures the company's continued independence.

Los Angeles | London | New Delhi | Singapore | Washington DC | Melbourne

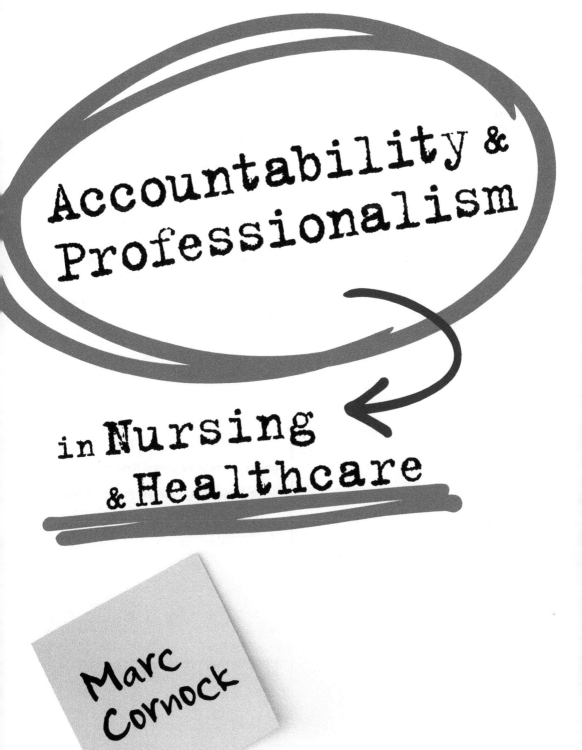

Accountability & Professionalism

in Nursing & Healthcare

Marc Cornock

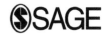

Los Angeles | London | New Delhi
Singapore | Washington DC | Melbourne

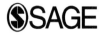

Los Angeles | London | New Delhi
Singapore | Washington DC | Melbourne

SAGE Publications Ltd
1 Oliver's Yard
55 City Road
London EC1Y 1SP

SAGE Publications Inc.
2455 Teller Road
Thousand Oaks, California 91320

SAGE Publications India Pvt Ltd
B 1/I 1 Mohan Cooperative Industrial Area
Mathura Road
New Delhi 110 044

SAGE Publications Asia-Pacific Pte Ltd
3 Church Street
#10-04 Samsung Hub
Singapore 049483

Editor: Laura Walmsley
Editorial assistant: Sahar Jamfar
Production editor: Nicola Marshall
Copyeditor: Christobel Colleen Hopman
Proofreader: Benny Willy Stephen
Marketing manager: Ruslana Khatagova
Cover design: Sheila Tong
Typeset by: TNQ Technologies

Library of Congress Control Number: 2022945319

British Library Cataloguing in Publication data

A catalogue record for this book is available from the British Library

ISBN 978-1-5297-7599-0
ISBN 978-1-5297-7600-3 (pbk)

Dedicated to Tina, the best 'sister' anyone could have.

And to Jane Bryant, the best CM any MC could have. Thank you for all you have done, and do, to make work more fun, and ensuring that I get it all done and on time (well mostly, but that's my fault as I am sure you will tell me 😊).

CONTENTS

DETAILED TABLE OF CONTENTS

LIST OF TABLES

ABOUT THE AUTHOR

Marc Cornock is an academic lawyer and Senior Lecturer in Healthcare Law in the Faculty of Wellbeing, Education and Language Studies, The Open University. Before joining the Faculty of Health and Social Care at The Open University, Marc was Senior Lecturer in Law at The Open University Law School and prior to that was Principal Lecturer and Academic Lead for Law in Health Care in the Faculty of Health and Social Work at the University of Plymouth.

During a professional career within healthcare, Marc undertook a master's degree in Medical Law and a PhD at Cardiff University Law School and studied undergraduate law at The Open University.

Marc's teaching interests lie in both general law and in health law. Marc has lectured on legal aspects of health care to various professional groups. His research focuses on the interface between the law and healthcare practice, and he has written extensively on this for professional and academic audiences. He is the author of *Key Questions in Healthcare Law and Ethics*, also published by SAGE Publications Ltd.

AUTHOR'S ACKNOWLEDGEMENTS

Although I am the named author, this book would not exist were it not for a group of individuals who have assisted me in its development from its initial conception through writing to its actual production. I would like to take this opportunity to formally say thank you to each and every one of them, including those anonymous reviewers who provided valuable feedback during its development stage.

To my colleagues and students who have shared the journey with me and discussed the concepts in this book, whether in a lecture or seminar or workshop or in the refectory. A heartfelt thank you for allowing me to share your thoughts and 'bounce' ideas off you and with you, whilst hopefully journeying together.

I would like to particularly mention Dr. Andrew Nichols who has been influential in the development of this book and has been more than generous with his time and advice. To say he is a lecturer extraordinaire does not do him justice. I can only wish I were one of his students.

I need to say a massive thank you to my family and friends. Perhaps I should have told you that I was writing the 'difficult second book' and that was why I was not always available: mea culpa and I am sorry. Thanks for putting up with my writing, again, and for allowing (or was it tolerating?) my disappearances as I had a sudden realisation about something that I wanted to write down, usually when I had no pen and paper or electronic method of making a note. Three family members deserve special mention, Tim Fielden for discussing the contents of this book and its format in the evening around the fire at Adam and Emma's wedding reception, and Adam and Emma Foxcroft for inviting me to the wedding where the discussion happened (outside of my own, it remains one of my favourite weddings to have attended!). The delay between the date of the wedding and that of the book's publication is entirely my fault and I don't hold any of the three of you responsible.

Sarah, if it were not for you this book would not exist and I cannot express my thanks adequately enough for all the support and encouragement you have given me throughout the whole planning and writing process.

Marc Cornock
West Yorkshire
August 2022

INTRODUCTION

This book is concerned with what it means to be accountable as a professional healthcare practitioner. It does this by reviewing what a professional is, what it means to be a professional working in healthcare and by examining the ways that a healthcare practitioner is accountable for their actions. It considers how healthcare practitioners need to work with others in teams, both within their own professional group and with practitioners from other professions, and how clinical decisions are made. It also examines how patient rights can be respected, and patent safety may be ensured. It concludes by addressing what may happen if things go wrong during the course of healthcare delivery.

This book may be a bit different to many you will pick up. So I have written this introduction to explain what it is about and the approach I have taken when writing it.

The subject matter of this book, professions and accountability, has interested me for some time. It was integral to aspects of my doctoral research which examined how healthcare practitioners are regulated. They are also subjects that I have taught to different groups of students for many years. Consequently, my understanding of the concepts in this book has developed during those teaching sessions and through discussion with colleagues who shared my interest in the subjects. During my teaching, it became apparent that different groups of healthcare practitioners shared the same anxieties and dilemmas regarding their practice and how they met their professional obligations, notably their accountability. Also, that I was being asked similar questions regardless of the student's area of practice or their level of experience. Over time, and through discussion with my fellow lecturers, a group of common questions emerged.

This book includes and answers those common questions.

Now a word about what the book is not. It is not a formal textbook on professionalism or accountability; it is not a dry list of questions with equally dry answers. I have endeavoured to make the answers simple and as interesting as possible so that you can get to the root of the problem quickly. This book covers the common questions that I have been asked about professionalism and accountability: the ones that you may want to ask, the ones that everyone assumes that everyone else knows.

It has been written so that it will be appropriate for all levels of healthcare practitioner from the learner, in the initial stages of their education, to the advanced practitioner who wishes to refresh their knowledge, or maybe learn something new.

What is unique about this book? It is based around a question and answer approach. If we were able to sit down and chat, this is what you may ask and how I would answer. The approach taken in each of the chapters is to avoid large chucks of indigestible material by using questions that ensure all the important information can be covered in the answer provided. Each chapter is structured but in a way that allows you to easily find what you may be looking for. There is no need for you to start at page 1 and read to the end, though feel free to do so if you want. You can go straight to the question you want answered and read that answer. Most of the answers are short(ish), although one or two are notably longer because of their complexity.

SOME 'HEALTH WARNINGS'

Throughout the book, the word 'patient' has been used as shorthand for clients, patients and individuals in receipt of care and treatment from healthcare practitioners. Similarly, 'healthcare practitioner' is used as shorthand for anyone who provides care, treatment, advice, counselling, guidance or in other ways meets the health and care needs of patients. It is used for all grades of practitioner and all professional groups. Where a law or guidance or policy refers to a specific practitioner group, for example nurse, this word will be used.

There is no index to this book, for two reasons. Firstly, the list of questions in the **Detailed Table of Contents** pages will hopefully assist you in finding the information you are looking for, as the questions are written in a manner that indicates what is addressed in the answer as well as being written in the language that they were asked. Secondly, having spent a large part of my life trying to find things in indexes, I have realised I don't find them that useful, as very often when I look something up, I find that the author has used a different word to the one I am using, and I can't find what I am looking for. I hope that the use of questions will prevent this happening to you. All the questions are either a direct question I have been asked during my teaching or a modified question to make the subject of the answer clearer.

If, for instance, you wanted to search for information on delegation you could look at the **Detailed Table of Contents** pages and search for the word, and in Chapter 4 you will see there is a question **What is delegation?** If you go to that question, you will find the information on delegation. I guess in many ways the **Detailed Table of Contents** is my substitute for an index!

Oh, the bold bit in the paragraph above. I need to explain that to you. Sometimes to answer a question I need to refer you to another question. To do that I will put the question you need to move to in bold. Of course, it's up to you if you do but it's my suggestion of where you may find additional information.

Some of the questions could usefully sit in one or of more of the chapters as they apply to several of the chapter themes. I discussed this with several groups of students and their location is where those students said they would commonly look for the information. Hopefully, they weren't a particularly odd bunch of students and it will be a logical location for you as well!

The structure of each chapter follows a familiar format. There is an introduction to what the chapter will discuss; a list of questions that will be addressed; the questions and answers; a summary of the main points; and a reference list.

The book may be thought of as having two parts. Part 1, which comprises Chapters 1 and 2, has the 'big word' chapters, the ones which explore the key concepts and lay the foundation for Part 2. Part 2 is all the remaining chapters. Chapters 3 through 7 build upon Chapters 1 and 2 and apply and develop the concepts found in them to specific areas and issues within professionalism and accountability. Part 2 may be seen as applying the concepts in Part 1. The chapters in Part 2 address the overall question of this book: what do I, as a healthcare practitioner, need to do to ensure that I am an accountable professional and how do I work with others for the safety of the patient?

MY APPROACH TO WRITING

In this book, I have adopted an informal chatty style of writing so that the information should feel related to the actual work that you do. The style I have used in this book is an extension of my teaching approach; I think that my students learn best when they are relaxed with the subject, hence the informal style to my writing. The answers I provide in this book are the answers I would provide to you if you asked the question in my lectures, seminars and workshops. In fact, they contain more information than there is usually time to cover in the teaching environment!

However, don't be fooled into thinking that the informal approach is superficial in its covering of subjects, or I am not serious about the subject or its consequences. I remain passionate about my subject and also my teaching of it. It is possible to be both serious about a subject but also to be informal and at times irreverent about it. The reason for the informal approach and use of questions is that it allows each subject to be divided into manageable chunks that are not dry and distant from the work you do. You could read through a chapter using the questions as your guide, or if you are looking for the answer to a specific problem, use the questions in the **Detailed Table of Contents** to determine where the answer will be found.

I hope that you find this book to be informative and interesting but also enjoyable. I welcome any comments you may have. I would be keen to hear if there is a question that you would have liked to have asked or something extra you would wish to be included in an answer. Let the publisher know, I am sure they will tell me.

Thanks for reading this far.

Marc

PROFESSIONALISM

Chapter 1 introduces the concept of professionalism in the healthcare context. It does this through considering what a profession is and what it means to be a professional and then applies this to the healthcare context. A discussion of morals, values and ethics then follows before examining what a professional issue is. Chapter 1 concludes by looking at how entry to the healthcare professions and the use of titles are issues of concern to the healthcare professions.

QUESTIONS COVERED IN CHAPTER 1

- What is a profession?
- Has the notion of professions remained consistent?
- What models and approaches have been used to distinguish a profession from other occupational groups?
- Does it matter if an occupation is a profession or not?
- What does it mean to be a professional?
- What is a healthcare professional?
- Is there a legal definition of healthcare professional?
- What are morals?
- What are ethics?
- What is the difference between morals and ethics?
- What are values?
- Do professional values differ from ethics?
- How do morals, ethics and professional values relate to being a professional?
- What ethical principles are relevant to healthcare practice?
- What is a professional issue?
- Why is pre-registration education a professional issue?
- Is it important to restrict the use of titles?

Q

What is a profession?

A

Talking about professions is something that is commonplace, but rarely is the term explained to check that there is common agreement about what is being discussed so that all involved are actually discussing the same entity.

Dictionaries generally define the word 'profession' in terms of an occupation that requires some form of learning or training leading to specialist (or professional) knowledge. There is also an acknowledgement that entry to the profession is controlled in some way so that it is not possible to just join the profession. Instead, there has to be a fulfilment of some form of entry requirement by the person seeking entry before entry to the profession is attained. There is usually also a requirement that the professional knowledge is used for the benefit of others.

Aligned with the need for training and education and the controlling of entry, a profession also has some form of identity. This identity is necessary to separate that particular group from another group.

For a profession to exist separate to a group of workers undertaking the same task, there has to be some form of body or organisation that can organise the activities of the profession. This body also needs to oversee the training and education of members, and potential members, of the profession, and allow entry to the profession for those who have the appropriate training and/or education.

This is neatly summarised by Freidson when he stated that a profession is '*an occupation that controls its own work, organised by a special set of institutions, sustained, in part, by a particular ideology of expertise and service*' (1994 at page 10).

Professions are not static. They do not come into being and stay the same, rather they grow and evolve organically throughout their existence according to the need and means of the society in which they function. This is part of the profession maintaining its professional identity and its relevance.

The relationship between a profession and society is very different to that between society and a group of occupations. The occupational group, or group of non-professional workers undertaking similar tasks, undertake their tasks according to the needs of those who control their work. A profession goes beyond organising its members to perform their role. The profession's relationship with the society it operates in allows it to work with that society to establish what it needs the profession to do, that is, how the aspect of society that is under the profession's remit can be best managed for the benefit of society. This is the so-called professional mandate where the profession controls the direction it takes for the benefit of society.

Q

Has the notion of professions remained consistent?

A

As can be expected by the fact that the question was asked, no, there has not been a consistent approach to what a profession is. Nor has there been a consistent number of professions since certain occupational groups were first recognised as professions.

In relation to the first profession, Bush and Cornock write that '*it is commonly agreed that the roots of professionalism can be found in the role of the church during the middle ages. At that time the church was practically the sole provider of services to the state and the general public at large. The main reason for this was that they had a near monopoly of learning and thus, the body of knowledge contained in their libraries. Due to this, the church provided most health care, welfare, the making and administration of law, as well as teaching* (1999, page 8)'.

As the church began to lose its influence and power in the latter part of the sixteenth century, it also lost its monopoly on the services it had been providing. Though change was not immediate in terms of recognition of other professions to take over the roles the church had. Macdonald (1995) notes that discussion of professions has been happening since the eighteenth century. The first national census occurred in 1841; at that time, the recognised professions were divinity, law and medicine. By the time of the 1881 national census, the number of professions had risen to 19 (Bush & Cornock, 1999).

As the definition of what a profession is changed, different occupational groups have risen to recognition as a profession since then. There have been several ways of determining what a profession is and what occupational groups need to 'achieve' to be seen as a profession. It is, therefore, the view within society at any given point in time that determines what a profession is and whether a particular occupational group is seen as a profession or not, and the number of professions that exist. This change in what is the prevalent view of a profession is what has resulted in the inconsistency around an occupational group achieving the status of becoming a profession.

The 1960s and 1970s saw an increase in discussion around the phenomena and criteria that distinguishes a profession from non-professional occupation groups (for instance, see Witz, 1992). During that time the traditional view of what constituted a profession changed, and various models, theoretical concepts and approaches were proposed to address who is and is not a profession.

Q **What models and approaches have been used to distinguish a profession from other occupational groups?**

A One of the major approaches to distinguish between professions and other occupational groups is that of the taxonomic approach. The taxonomic approach is based on the theory that a profession is in possession of some unique characteristics that set it apart from other occupational groups, and these characteristics give it an increased importance within society.

In the taxonomic approach, there is an interplay between possession of the necessary characteristics and how society views that group. For Saks, '*professions both possess some unique characteristics which set them apart from other occupations and play a positive and important role in the division of labour in society*' (1983 at page 2).

Within the taxonomic approach there are two main variations: the trait and the functionalist.

The trait view holds that there are certain traits or attributes that *'are held to represent the core features of professional occupations'* (Saks, 1983 at page 2). As may be imagined, even among those who favoured the trait variation of the taxonomic approach, there was not consensus on what these traits were. Some commentators held that there were a few key traits, such as Goode (1960) who believed there were only two core characteristics (a service orientation and training in a unique body of knowledge). While others, such as Millerson (1964), held that there were as many as 23 separate traits that had to be fulfilled for an occupational group to be considered a profession.

Despite the lack of consensus as to how many traits there should be and what all these are, there is some commonality that can be identified in the various trait views. The trait view usually includes the following as attributes needed to become a profession:

- A code of ethics or accepted behaviours
- Authority to act provided by those the profession serves
- Autonomous practice
- Being able to set standards for education and training
- Body of theoretical knowledge
- Competence testing
- Controlling entry to the profession and the granting of a licence to practise
- Having the power to remove those no longer able to practise
- Maintaining a list of those licensed to practise
- Power to sanction members of the profession
- Professional culture that is maintained (and reinforced) by the profession
- Service to society
- Set minimum periods of education and training

Those within the taxonomic approach that proposed a functionalist view held that that is a 'contract' being the profession and society in which the profession performs a vital function for society and in return is rewarded with an increased standing within society and occupational privileges. These privileges would normally include the attributes in the list above.

The functionalist view, therefore, asks not what attributes the profession claims to have but what distinctive role does the profession have in maintaining society. In essence, what is it that the profession does that means society would not be able to function without it?

Another view on professions is that of the neo-Weberian view of social closure. From this viewpoint, professions are not about having particular traits or function in society but rather is concerned with occupational groups operating to restrict the ability of outsiders to enter the occupation. In this way, the profession acts as a control that exists solely to maintain the status and associated privileges and benefits of the profession but only for those who are members of the profession by excluding others from undertaking that occupation.

More recently, these views have been seen to be limiting, and hybrid views of profession have been proposed which 'borrow' from several of the earlier approaches. In this way a profession is seen as having both a function in society as well as fulfilling specific traits including seeking to exclude individuals from its occupation but only until they have attained the necessary skills, knowledge and competence to join the profession.

Q Does it matter if an occupation is a profession or not?

A It may seem an odd question to ask 'does it matter if a particular occupation is a profession or not' in a book on professions. But it is a valid question to raise because it means we can address whether there is a tangible benefit to the profession, the person within the profession and/or society itself.

The short answer to this question is yes, in modern society it does matter.

For society, having professions operate within it means that part of the function of that society can be left to the profession to operationalise and regulate. Thereby reducing the burden on society while still maintaining the service that society needs to function.

For the profession, there still exists the status and associated privileges and benefits that come with being classed as a profession within any particular society. The most important of these privileges may be said to be the ability to self-regulate in terms of being able to set its own standards for entry and for continued membership of the profession.

For the members of the profession, the reason it matters is because of how professionals are treated in comparison to non-professional workers. Non-professional workers can be seen as working to a form of master and servant arrangement whereby the 'master' provides direction to the worker as to what work they need to do and when and where. There will also be, to a greater or lesser extent, a degree of the master controlling how the worker undertakes their work.

The professional on the other hand is treated in a very different way to the non-professional worker. Although the majority of professionals may work for one employer, their status means that they have a greater degree of autonomy over their role and the use of their expertise. It is the professional who decides their sphere of competence.

Q What does it mean to be a professional?

A If professions exist (see **What is a profession?** and **Has the notion of professions remained consistent?**) then by default there have to be professionals, that is, members of that profession. The aim of this question is to see what the difference is between someone working at the level of a professional as opposed to someone working at the level of the non-professional.

To be a professional in modern society is not an insignificant undertaking. It is not a simple step of being accepted for and becoming a member of a defined occupational group that has achieved the status of a profession because there are all the challenges and obligations that exist with that professional status (see **What is regulation?** and **How does regulation affect the healthcare practitioner?** for further discussion of these points), as well as the benefits that come with being a professional.

In **Does it matter if an occupation is a profession or not?** it was stated that being a professional means the individual has a greater degree of autonomy over their role, a discretionary element in how they perform their role but also in when and whether to perform that role. It is the professional who knows if their expertise is required or not. In order to exercise their autonomy, the professional has to demonstrate that they have acquired the necessary knowledge, skill and ability to be considered a professional in the first place but also that they have maintained that knowledge, skill and ability so that they remain current within their sphere of practise.

Being a professional means a commitment to maintaining and advancing competence (competence is defined and discussed in **What is clinical competence?**).

This professional behaviour, the acquisition of knowledge and skills and abilities to be able to perform their role, may be one of the fundamental aspects of being a professional in modern society. Along with the commitment to its maintenance and development.

Beaty has proposed that being a professional is not a simple process and certainly not a, 'is or isn't' situation, rather she sees a continuum of professional behaviour. For Beaty *'skill is acquired through routine practice and decision making. Thus, for the novice, experiential knowledge is small and decisions will be tentative and rule bound to avoid mistakes. After some experience the application of rules becomes more automatic and there are fewer surprises in practice. Thus longer-term goals become visible and procedures are applied routinely and with less anxiety. The expert moves beyond rules to more 'intuitive' action where a deep understanding of context informs a view of what is routine and what is novel'* (2000 at page 18).

It is the acknowledgement that the professional has a professional behaviour ethic that means society is prepared to invest in their professional mandate. It is this professional mandate that allows the professional and, in turn, the profession to inform society of how the aspect of society that the profession operates in can be best managed. Through the professional mandate, the professional has a great responsibility than an occupational worker. The professional has a responsibility to inform society of when something is wrong or not working and needs to be changed and to provide a solution as to how it can be improved for the benefit of all in that society, not just the professional themselves.

What is a healthcare professional?

It needs to be recognised that although the term 'healthcare professional' is being used here for various groups of professional, in reality, the different professionals within the healthcare setting are not a single group but rather comprise different professional groupings. Each of the different professions would clearly and succinctly point out the differences between themselves and any of the other professions which work in the healthcare setting.

Healthcare professional is being used here for simplicity so as not to have to refer to (in alphabetical order) chiropodists and podiatrists, dieticians, doctors, midwives, nurses, occupational therapist, paramedics, physiotherapists, radiographers, speech therapists etc. each time a question is being answered. Though equally, it has to be recognised that there are similarities between the different professions working within healthcare which is why they are being discussed together.

Time to move on before we get bogged down in a discussion on the boundaries between the healthcare professions and the blurring of boundaries that has occurred in recent times!

The healthcare professional has to fulfil the definition of being a professional and then to somehow apply this to the healthcare context in some shape or form. The definition of what a professional is will not be discussed any further in this particular answer but see **What does it mean to be a professional?** for a discussion of what this entails.

To be a healthcare professional, the individual has to be connected to healthcare through their work. Although working in healthcare alone cannot simply be enough otherwise it would not be possible to differentiate the healthcare professional from the healthcare worker.

But just one minute, what do we mean by connected to healthcare: how are they connected and what is healthcare? Have a go at defining what you think healthcare means in terms of deciding if someone is a healthcare worker/professional or not.

Determining what constitutes healthcare in this context is both difficult and easy. It is easy because it is obvious: healthcare is anything that affects a patient. It is short, neat and does what it says on the tin. True the healthcare service consists of a myriad of different occupational groups of workers who may not at first sight be seen as healthcare professionals or workers but who do undertake roles that affect patients and so based on this simple definition would in fact be healthcare professionals or workers. For instance: the cook, the cleaner, the driver who brings the supplies to the hospital, the chief accountant who ensures that there is money to buy the necessary supplies and pay the staff. All work in healthcare but are all healthcare workers? This is why defining healthcare is difficult.

Maybe it would be easier to recognise that there are various occupational groups working within a healthcare setting but not all of these directly affect patients. Only those occupations that directly affect patients would be classified as healthcare workers as opposed to workers in a healthcare setting.

We would need to define what we mean by directly affect but we could say that patients are only directly affected by things that are undertaken by someone directly for the patient's benefit and that the patient is involved in. Some form of direct patient contact. Using this definition, the cook and the driver and the chief accountant all lose their status of healthcare worker/professional, but what of the cleaner?

There is another issue with this particular definition that can be summarised as when is a nurse not a nurse (feel free to substitute nurse with the healthcare occupational group of your choice). Imagine a nurse, registered with the Nursing and Midwifery Council (registration is discussed in **How does registration relate to being a professional?** and the role of the Nursing and Midwifery Council is outlined in **How does regulation affect the healthcare practitioner?**) working in a clinical area having direct contact with their patients. At this point, the definition we have put forward is great and we would all agree that nurse is a healthcare worker/professional. After a number of years in clinical practice, the nurse decides to pursue a career in nurse education. Eventually they end up in a department of nursing in a university, teaching student nurses. They no longer have any direct patient contact, although their students do.

Is this nurse a healthcare worker/professional under our definition? The key criteria was to have some direct patient contact which they no longer have. So, no, they can't be seen as a healthcare worker/professional at this point in their career. The same may be said for those healthcare workers/professionals who move into research or management, anywhere where they no longer have direct patient contact.

What if the nurse who has moved their focus of practice into education still maintains their registration with the Nursing and Midwifery Council? As far as the definition goes at the point at which they case to have direct patient contact, the definition no longer classifies them as healthcare workers/professionals. The Nursing and Midwifery Council would in effect be allowing non-healthcare workers/professionals to register with them, a ludicrous situation. Obviously the definition is not as useful as we thought.

Another definition that could be used is that a healthcare worker/professional is someone who can deliver healthcare to a patient. This changes the focus from using the patient as the focus of healthcare, so those who have no patient contact are excluded from being seen as healthcare workers/professional, to those who have the ability but may not necessarily use it directly with patients, rather they have an indirect effect on patients through their research or teaching of others.

This definition would exclude those that most people who probably not see as healthcare workers/professional, the cook, the cleaner, the driver and the chief accountant but includes those who have no direct patient contact such as the nurse researcher or nurse lecturer.

The only thing we now need to do is to decide what 'can deliver healthcare' means. One way of looking at this is to say that those who have undertaken a recognised qualification to practise in a specific healthcare field, such as midwifery or physiotherapy, can deliver healthcare to patients. The preparation in attaining the qualification is what prepares them for delivering healthcare to a patient.

'AN ASIDE ON STUDENTS AND BEING A PROFESSIONAL'

Considering the discussion above, can you be a professional while you are a student on a programme of study that leads to a recognised healthcare qualification?

(Continued)

> You can certainly exhibit the behaviours of a professional and work to professional standards. However, if the professional is someone who has achieved the recognised qualification, until you have achieved it, you would not be able to call yourself a healthcare professional.
>
> This is why this book uses the term 'healthcare practitioner', because it includes healthcare workers, healthcare professionals *and* healthcare students, as all are affected by issues of professionalism and accountability, even if some are more affected than others.

To summarise: a healthcare professional is someone who works with or for patients after achieving a recognised qualification to practise in a specific healthcare field, is competent (see What is clinical competence and **What does it mean to be a professional?**) to undertake their area of practice and also has a degree of autonomy or independence in how their perform their practice (see **What does it mean to be a professional?**). Anyone else who works with or for the benefit of patients is a healthcare worker and not a healthcare professional.

Q

A

Is there a legal definition of a healthcare professional?

Short answer, sort of.

Many Acts of Parliament, and other forms of legislation, mention healthcare professionals. Most either provide a definition or clarify what they mean by healthcare professional or make reference to other legislation that provides this clarification. However, the clarification or definition is not what we might expect.

Rather than provide a full definition of what a healthcare professional is (as defined in **What is a healthcare professional?**), the legislation states that a healthcare professional is someone who is currently on one of the professional registers maintained by the statutory healthcare regulatory bodies (see **How does regulation affect the healthcare practitioner?** for the remit of the statutory healthcare regulator bodies).

Registration is the mechanism by which the healthcare professions control entry to the profession (control of entry to the profession being a requirement of having recognition as a profession, see **What is a profession?**), see **How does registration relate to being a professional?** for a discussion of the professional registers.

Using this legislative definition of a healthcare professional, those who are not registered fail on the first principle and would instead be seen as healthcare workers, provided they fulfil the other criteria discussed in **What is a healthcare professional?** regarding working in healthcare.

If the definition of a healthcare professional has to include being registered with a professional regulatory body, the definition of a healthcare professional proposed in **What is a healthcare professional?** can be revised to be someone who:

- works with or for patients after achieving a recognised qualification to practise in a specific healthcare field
- has current registration (**How does registration relate to being a professional?** outlines the purpose of registration and what it means for a healthcare practitioner) with one of the healthcare regulatory bodies (the role of the regulatory bodies is outlined in **How does regulation affect the healthcare practitioner?**)
- is competent (for a discussion of competence see **What is clinical competence?** provides a discussion of competence) to undertake their area of practice
- has a degree of accountability (discussed in several questions in **Chapter 2**) for their practice
- has a degree of autonomy or independence in how they perform their practice

Again, anyone else who works with or for the benefit of patients is a healthcare worker and not a healthcare professional.

What are morals?

Morals are not something that we can choose to have or not. Neither are they something that are imposed upon us but instead are an innate part of each of us. Morals are personal to the individual. They do not arrive fully formed but develop over time to act as a system of checks and balances upon our behaviour. They can develop from an individuals' personal experience and their religious beliefs and also how they view society and their place within it.

Morals relate to how a particular person lives their life and what they believe is right and wrong. As such, morals can be thought of as an individual internal belief system. Morals are sometimes referred to as a moral compass. This is a useful analogy as like a compass they guide the direction in which a person may go, only this is not a direction of travel but direction of what to do when faced with a dilemma or decision.

Morals are the principles that a person uses to guide them in making choices in their life.

What are ethics?

Ethics are, when reduced to its fundamentals, a system of beliefs about right and wrong. It is a system for understanding human behaviour and why a particular individual may act in a particular way in a given set of circumstances.

Ethics are more formalised than morals (see **What are morals?**), but like morals, they relate to decision-making and concepts of right and wrong.

Various ethics theories have developed with two main theories traditionally being proposed for healthcare, these being deontology and utilitarianism.

There were two ethical theories that were traditionally taught and considered to be relevant to healthcare practitioners and to healthcare itself. These are Deontology and Utilitarianism. Here we will look at both of these theories in the way that they were presented, that is, as a binary approach to ethics: something was approached through either a deontological or utilitarian outlook.

DEONTOLOGY

Deontology literally means the study of duty. It arises from the Greek for duty, 'Deon'. As an ethical theory, it can be traced back to the work of Immanuel Kant, a Prussian philosopher working in the mid to late 1700s. Kant's philosophical theory is grounded in what he termed the 'categorical imperative'.

A categorical imperative is something that has an intrinsic nature about it that is good. No external validation is needed to make them good. For humans to be morally good, they have to follow all categorical imperatives. Therefore, a categorical imperative becomes a selfless act; it is something that has to be done because of a duty or obligation to do so. Duty or obligation are key underlying features of deontology as Kant believed that if someone acts without there being a duty to do so, there is no moral value to that action.

One aspect of the categorical imperative is that individuals should always act as if their action was to become a universal ethical law for others to follow, that is, to act without any personal motive.

Someone who acted according to deontological ethics would do so because they felt they had a duty or obligation to do so. They would have no free will in the choice of action but would feel compelled to act in a certain way. Thus, actions can be classified as being good or bad according to the reasons behind the act. Failing to act when there is a duty to do so would be seen as behaving unethically.

Therefore, for deontologists, clear duties and obligations exist in given situations. For instance, the healthcare practitioner who is off-duty but comes across someone who requires their assistance would have a clear duty to act for the benefit of the individual rather than themselves (see **Are there any special considerations in the duty of care or standard of care?**).

In this way, codes of practice can be said to have a deontological ethical basis as they require the individual subject to them to act in certain ways because of their duty or obligations (see **What is a code of conduct?** and **Do codes of conduct have legal status?** for a discussion of codes of conduct and their use). Indeed, the Health and Care Professions Council (HCPC) 'Standards of conduct, performance and ethics' (Health and Care Professions Council, 2016) actually begins with the words '*your duties as a registrant*' (title page). Each of the ten standards that make up the 'code' then begins with the words '*you must*'. The Nursing and Midwifery Council (NMC) code has a similar approach, with its introduction stating that '*The code contains the professional standards that registered nurses, midwives and nursing associates must uphold*' (Nursing and Midwifery Council, 2018 page 2). Similar to the HCPC code, each of the 25 standards in the NMC code start with '*To achieve this you must*'. It is only after the duty has been stated do the codes provide any guidance as to how you, the healthcare practitioner, who has to use and follow them, may achieve the duty.

When considering how to act in any situation, the person acting according to a deontological ethical perspective would ask, 'What is my clear duty in this situation?' Not, 'What should I do?', or 'What do I want to do?' but 'What do I have to do?'

UTILITARIANISM

Utilitarianism developed through the late 1700s and the early 1800s and was generally influenced by two British philosophers, Jeremy Bentham and John Stuart Mill. It is also known as consequentialism (for reasons that will soon become apparent).

Compared with deontology, utilitarianism is said to be a much easier ethical theory to understand. Its basic premise is that an act should be based on the premise of maximising utility and minimising worthlessness: or, to put it another way, doing the greatest good and the least harm. Thus, any action is judged not by it being a universal right or wrong as in deontology but on the outcome it produces. The consequences of the action are the key aspect of any act in utilitarianism/consequentialism.

Those actions that result in more good than harm are seen as being more ethically desirable in utilitarianism.

Other ways of looking at utility and worthlessness are pleasure or happiness and pain or suffering. Accordingly, utilitarianism is often referred to as 'the greatest happiness principle'.

However, rather than concentrating on pleasure at the level of the individual, the utilitarian theory concentrates upon the greatest happiness for the greatest number of people. If I were to do something that gives me pleasure but causes pain for more people than it provides happiness, this would go against utilitarian ideologies. However, if I can gain pleasure or happiness from doing an act which also gives others more pleasure than pain, this would be in accordance with utilitarian theory.

Therefore, when considering any act, the individual must consider the outcomes in terms of the number of individuals it affects, and the type of effect that it will have upon them, as well as the length and severity of that effect. You should act to cause the greatest good or happiness for the greatest number of people for the longest period of time.

There are two types of utilitarian ethical thinking: the act utilitarian and the rule utilitarian. The act utilitarian considers the nature of an act and the consequences that follow from undertaking the act, or from not undertaking the act, and chooses the decision, doing or not doing the act, that results in the greatest happiness. The rule utilitarian, on the other hand, considers what the outcome would be if the rule, whether to act or not, was always followed. If always following the rule would produce more happiness than always not following the rule, then the rule is followed, and vice versa. The rule utilitarian may be seen to be a cross between the act utilitarian and the deontologist, in that they act for the greatest good but according to a general rule and not on an individually thought out basis.

Q **What is the difference between morals and ethics?**

A Morals and ethics are closely related in that both related to notions of right and wrong or good and bad and both affect how a person may act in any given situation.

Both morals and ethics assist individuals in making decisions that are right for them according to the ecocide system they operate within.

Whereas morals are an internal system of beliefs that are unique to the individual, ethics are more concerned with accepted behaviour in a group of individuals. If morals are personal beliefs, then ethics are shared beliefs and norms of acceptable behaviour.

In the same way that morals are unique to an individual, ethics are unique to the group or society that they apply to.

Q **What are values?**

A At its simplest level, a value is the worth attributed to something, not necessarily monetary, or the importance that should be attached to it.

Cuthbert and Quallington state that '*values are particular kinds of beliefs that are concerned with the worth or value of an idea or behaviour and are important in guiding our actions, our judgements, our behaviour and our attitudes towards others*' (2017 at page 5).

There is a relationship between morals (see **What are morals?**) and values. This is because a person's beliefs about what is right and wrong will affect how they perceive something. For instance, someone who does not believe in the ownership of property may attribute less value to a car than someone who does not have the same moral belief. Similarly, someone who has the moral belief that lying is always wrong will probably place more importance on truth telling than someone who does not share that belief. It is the value placed on the thing by the individual that is important.

Values can apply to tangible objects such as property, or to more abstract concepts such whether a particular piece of art is important, or the ideological as with whether euthanasia should be legalised.

Values are not an objective standard because the beliefs of one person may place the value of X higher or lower than the next person. Though values exist not just at the level of the individual and can exist at the level of a group or at a societal level.

According to Goodman and Clemow, '*one way to uncover them* [values] *is to note what is respected or honoured within a group*' (2010 at page 70).

Professions can be said to have shared values which are seen in the behaviours that are expected of the members of that profession by those within the profession, and by those outside of the profession as well.

Professional values can be seen to be behind the statement in **What does it mean to be a professional?** that professional behaviour involves the acquisition of knowledge and skills and abilities by the professional to be able to perform their role. This is because it is the professional value(s) shared by the profession's members that results in the behaviours exhibited.

Shared professional values are therefore a vital element of professionalism and being a professional means aligning oneself to the values of that profession, at least in part.

Q Do professional values differ from ethics?

A A brief recap from **What are ethics?** and **What are values?** before we answer this question. Ethics are a system for understanding human behaviour and provide a formalised basis for action in a given situation, whereas values are the worth or importance applied to something, for instance, an object or a concept.

As well as the advantages in using ethical theory to support decision-making, there are also limitations in their use. Cornock (2021) notes the following as some of the limitations of deontology and utilitarianism:

DEONTOLOGY

- Lacks emotional element of human behaviour
- Does not allow for free-will of individuals
- Concentrates on performing a duty rather than the consequence of the action performed

UTILITARIANISM

- Striving for the greatest happiness can result in poor outcomes at the individual level.
- Individual rights can be subjugated for the greater happiness.
- Predicting outcomes and the greatness happiness can result in difficulty in deciding between two actions.
- What is happiness or a good outcome is subjective.
- While the intent may be to cause happiness, the outcome may be the opposite.

Because of the limitations on the traditional ethical theories and their binary approach, particularly when seen from a healthcare perspective, there has been a move away from them and from the notion of a single ethical theory that answers all ethical queries. Cornock states that *'rather than there being a right decision based on a specific ethical theory or framework, a healthcare practitioner can use ethical principles to guide their decision making'* (2021 at pages 11–12). The ethical principles just mentioned are discussed in **What ethical principles are relevant to healthcare practice?**

These ethical principles mentioned by Cornock are based in ethical virtues or values. These can be used at the individual or group level and represent what that person or group believes to underpin decision-making. In this way, it is the values of the person or group that set their ethical principles.

So while there is a fundamental difference between ethics and values, in practice, particularly in healthcare practice, there is an overlap in how ethics and values have resulted in the development of the beliefs of the various healthcare professions and what value they place on certain behaviours and which behaviours they value more highly than others. This overlap is demonstrated in the professional values that are put forth by the various professions.

Q

How do morals, ethics and professional values relate to being a professional?

A

As we saw in **What is the difference between morals and ethics?**, there is a relationship between a person's moral beliefs and ethical principles in that both involve notions of right and wrong, good and bad. Equally both are concerned with how someone acts in a given situation.

While discussing **What are values?** it was noted that morals and values are connected because an individual's personal beliefs will affect the value they place on something, be that a tangible object or an abstract concept.

So at the level of the individual, the relationship between morals, ethic and values can be seen. At the level of the profession, in discussing **Do professional values differ from ethics?**, it was stated that despite the difference between ethics and values, both have contributed to the beliefs that the profession puts forward and the professional values that it holds and requires members of that profession to adhere to.

Indeed, instead of there being a difference between ethics and values in the professional context, professional values can be seen to be a way of utilising two distinct ways of looking at the world to develop a shared belief system and a shared basis for decision-making.

For the individual, separate from any personal beliefs and values that they may have, if they are a professional, they will also need to engage with the shared belief system of the profession to which they belong.

The shared belief system is a set of beliefs that guides the professional through the many decisions they have to make throughout their professional lives, based on the values attributed to those shared beliefs, as well as the sorts of behaviour they are expected to exhibit.

It may be simplest to think of the professional values of a particular profession as the guide that the profession offers to its members. For the healthcare professions, this is most often communicated in the form of codes of conduct (these are discussed in **What is a code of conduct?**). In this way, professional values are the ethical principles that the profession wants the members of the profession to exhibit in their professional work.

Cornock (2021) is of the opinion that ethical principles used by healthcare professionals and for healthcare practice arose because *'because no single ethical theory is suitable for all healthcare dilemmas'* (at page 12).

Within healthcare the ethical principles that are common to the various healthcare professions in guiding the practice of their members and for their members to use as part of ethical decision-making are:

- Autonomy
- Beneficence
- Non-maleficence
- Justice

These four ethical principles are explored further in **What ethical principles are relevant to healthcare practice?**

Answering this question has taken us from morals, through ethics, to values, to professional values. The professional is affected by them because they are expected to practise their profession in accordance with the professional values set out by the profession. These professional values provide the basis for the professional's behaviour as well as the underlying principles that guide their professional decision-making.

The individual professional who does not adhere to the shared belief system of their profession, by practising according to the profession's values, may find themselves acting outside of the profession's norm for behaviour and therefore at risk of censure or even expulsion from the profession.

What ethical principles are relevant to healthcare practice?

Beauchamp and Childress (2013) have proposed the use of ethical principles to assist healthcare practitioners in their ethical decision-making and guide their practice. These are: autonomy, beneficence, non-maleficence and justice.

AUTONOMY

Autonomy comes from the Greek for self-law or self-rule. It refers to being able to make decisions for oneself. To be autonomous, the individual has to be able to make decisions that are not coerced or subject to the will of others.

Respecting a person's autonomy is a key principle in both ethical thinking and the law. For a healthcare practitioner, who may be seen as someone in the position of authority with specialised knowledge and skills, to respect a person's autonomy means treating the person as an individual; respecting their ability to make decisions for themselves; providing them with information to allow them to make decisions; obtaining consent before attempting any procedure or treatment; respecting the person's confidentiality and adopting a professional approach to the person.

The opposite of respecting autonomy is paternalism, thinking that you, as the expert practitioner, know better than the patient. It is likely that you will know more about the art and science of being a healthcare practitioner and about healthcare practice; however, it is highly unlikely that you will know more than the patient about what their best interests are and how it is served. Healthcare practice is a partnership between you, as the practitioner, and the patient. Only then can the patient be autonomous.

Only a competent person (see **What is meant by competence?** for a discussion of what competence means and its relevance in healthcare and for a discussion of how healthcare practitioners can assess a patient's competence see **How is competence assessed?**) can be truly autonomous. This is because, if someone is unable to make decisions for themselves, they cannot be autonomous. However, it may be possible for a person to have autonomy with regard to certain aspects of their life and to be non-autonomous in others. For instance, to have autonomy over when they receive treatment but not over the type of treatment offered.

BENEFICENCE

Beneficence refers to doing good. For the healthcare practitioner, beneficence is related to promoting the wellbeing of the patient. Doing things that are of a benefit to the patient, undertaking procedures and treatment that serve the patient's best interests.

A problem arises in determining what is in the patient's best interests. The obvious answer is to ask the patient. Yet what would be the outcome if the healthcare practitioner wants to undertake a procedure that they believe to be in the patient's best interests, but the patient refuses it? Does the concept of the patient's autonomy override the healthcare practitioner's duty to be beneficent? This issue is addressed throughout this book. For now, it is sufficient to say that a healthcare practitioner is not doing good if they override a patient's rights, such as their right to autonomy.

NON-MALEFICENCE

Non-maleficence is related to the concept of '*primum non nocere*', which literally means first do no harm. The concept proposes that, whatever else you do, you should not harm your patient through your actions; therefore, doing nothing may be better than acting inappropriately and thereby causing harm. It is often thought of as being the same or similar to beneficence. However, the two are quite separate principles.

To act in a non-maleficent way, the healthcare practitioner has to ensure that they know the risks associated with the treatments and procedures they perform, when to perform them and when not, so that they do not cause harm to a patient through unnecessary treatment.

The challenge with both non-maleficence and beneficence is in making the judgement between not doing harm and doing good. I am often asked which is more important, to do good or to do no harm. I would argue that, if you don't do good, you have not left the patient worse off than before you didn't do anything; whereas if you fail to do no harm, you have in fact harmed the patient. By failing to do your non-maleficent duty, you cause harm; by failing to do your beneficent duty, the patient does not suffer.

JUSTICE

Justice as an ethical principle is related to fairness. There are different types of justice. One example is distributive justice which is concerned with the fair distribution of resources; another is rights based justice which relates to respecting the rights of individuals.

In the healthcare context, justice can refer to the obligation of treating individuals according to their need rather than any other criteria, to be just in the allocation of resources, including your skill, time and knowledge. It can also be concerned with providing justice to the wider society in not wasting the resource you have by treating those who are not in need of your skills.

Resource allocation is often cited as an aspect of justice in healthcare. How can a finite amount of resource be allocated fairly among all those in need if there is not enough to satisfy demand? This raises questions about whether it would be ethically right to withhold treatment from those with self-inflicted injuries, for instance, those who drink, fall down and injure themselves.

It could be argued that to do so would be in the interests of society by protecting a scarce resource; the alternative argument is that justice served by treating all those who require treatment, regardless of how they came to need that treatment. The question essentially reduces to whether justice should serve individuals or society. In reality, patients in the National Health Service are treated according to clinical need.

Q

What is a professional issue?

A

Ever seen a book which has 'professional issues' as a part of its title and wondered what exactly the book will contain? I have. Very often you can have a good guess at some of the content, but some usually flummox me either because I did not expect an issue to be included or because I expected an issue to be included and it wasn't.

A part of the problem is that different professions have different professional issues and what is a major issue for one profession may not even be seen as an issue by another profession in an unrelated area of practice. Although it is to be expected that professions in closely related areas of practice, such as those whose focus is on healthcare delivery, will share at least some professional issues.

There may not be consensus as to what professional issues different professions have, but there is a shared understanding of what a professional issue is.

The professional issues that a particular profession have are related to its professional values (see **What are values?** and **How do morals, ethics and professional values relate to being a professional?**). What a profession values will be instrumental in determining what it sees as an important issue that is worthy of its time and effort in addressing.

Some of the issues that a profession recognises as being important to it will be those that affect its members, or those that the professions serves. For the healthcare professions, this will be patients and also wider society which is affected if overall health is poor or healthcare provision is not sufficient to meet its needs. Therefore, issues that affect patients and their access to healthcare and issues that affect parts of society are professional issues for the professions with members practising within healthcare.

Thus, the healthcare professions will have many professional issues in common and may work together on addressing several of these, for instance, the level of provision of healthcare within specific population groups.

While there is commonality in the professional issues addressed by the healthcare professions, there may be difference in the level of importance they attach to a particular professional issue or the way in which they see to address it. There are also differences in the professional issues identified by professions that share a common area of practice. The reason for these differences in identification of issue and approach to addressing them is that the different professions have different professional values and different, albeit related, areas of practice. After all, if the professions fully shared their professional values and areas of practice, they would not be different professions (see **What is a profession?**).

For instance, professions A, B and C may all share how low income affects the health of individuals as a professional issue and seek a common approach to addressing this. They may all see workload as a professional issue but approach this in different ways, according to the needs of the members of their respective professions.

Yet only professions B and C may see expansion of the area of their clinical practice as a professional issue and only profession B may see relationships between them and other healthcare professionals as a professional issue that needs their attention.

In summary, a professional issue is an issue that affects the professional values of the profession, either because it affects it members directly, or affects the way in which the professionals in the profession undertake their practice or the area of their practice, or it affects those the profession serves, or it affects the way that the profession operates and governs itself.

Q
A

Why is pre-registration education a professional issue?

As a professional issue is an issue that is of concern to the profession because it in some way relates to the values of that profession (see **What is a professional issue?**), pre-registration education is a common shared professional issue among the healthcare professions.

The reason why pre-registration education is a common professional issue among the healthcare professions is that it goes to the core of professionalism. At their core professions have a set of shared values and agreement as to what constitutes professional behaviour (see **What does it mean to be a professional?** and **What are values?**). By influencing, and/or controlling, and/or regulating the preparation of those individuals who will become members of the profession through the requirements of pre-registration education, the profession is able to instil its professional values at the very beginning of the individual's journey to becoming a member of the profession.

Pre-registration education is also a way of gaining respect for the profession and its members via public recognition of the robustness of the preparation of members for the profession. As Montgomery states *'membership of the profession should indicate a level of training and expertise which enables the public to rely on the skill of the practitioner'* (2003 at page 133).

If it were felt that members of a particular profession were not adequately trained for their future roles, the profession may find that responsibility for preparation of their future members was removed from their remit.

Maintaining a degree of input into the preparation of future members by a profession ensures that a particular profession is able to influence and protect the curriculum so that what is taught covers the needs of the groups that the profession serves. Additionally, the profession is able to prepare future members for the roles that it believes are needed and will be needed in the future.

Pre-registration education, in addition to being a mechanism of exposing prospective members of a profession to that profession's professional values, is also a way of excluding those individuals who do not adhere to those professional values during their initial education.

The education of prospective members of a profession as professional issue is not a new phenomenon. Indeed, the General Medical Council was originally established in 1858 as the General Council of Medical Education and Registration of the United Kingdom.

Pre-registration education is a way of maintaining the profession's status and in ensuring the professional values of the profession, as well as preparing future members of the profession for their future roles. As such it is a key professional issue for professions.

Q **Is it important to restrict the use of titles?**

A The title that someone uses says a lot about them and a lot of what can be expected from them, hence the desire by professions to protect the titles of their members and restrict their use to members of that profession.

Professions want society and the people they serve to know who they can trust within the area of the profession's practice. That if someone is, for example, a physiotherapist, they can expect them to be competent in physiotherapy but also to have the professional values associated with the physiotherapy profession.

Protection of titles is now generally entrusted to regulatory bodies, particularly in healthcare, on behalf of the professions (**How does regulation affect the healthcare practitioner?** discusses the protection of titles by the regulatory bodies).

If someone uses a title that they are not entitled to use, they will be committing a criminal offence, with the possibility of an unlimited fine on conviction.

One of the problems with protecting titles is what title should be protected? Consider the following list of common titles used within healthcare and see which you think are protected titles:

- Chiropodist
- Dental nurse
- Dietician
- Doctor
- Midwife
- Nurse
- Paramedic
- Physiotherapist
- Therapeutic radiographer

The actual protected titles are as follows:

- Chiropodist
- Dental nurse
- Dietician
- Registered Medical Practitioner (rather than doctor)
- Midwife
- Registered Nurse (not just the title nurse)
- Paramedic
- Physiotherapist
- Therapeutic radiographer

If a title is not one that is protected, such as doctor or nurse, anyone can use it without fear of criminal conviction. Which is why there are sometimes calls for certain titles to receive the same protection as other titles used in healthcare such as paramedic or physiotherapist.

Generally, there are two reasons why a specific title is not protected. Firstly, because there is a protected title association with that particular occupation that fulfils the need of restricting entry to the profession as with registered nurse for nurses. Secondly, restricting the use of the title to those members of the particular profession would pose more problems than it solves. For instance, with the title doctor, there are many individuals who have a perfect entitlement to use the title other than those who are medical practitioners. Indeed, the title doctor was originally, and remains, an academic qualification and was used in medicine as an honorary title initially. Whereas with the title nurse there are many occupations which have nurse or a derivative of it in their title that are not associated with the nursing profession, for example, dental nurse, nursery nurse and veterinary nurse.

What would happen to those who use the title doctor or nurse but are not registered medical practitioners or registered nurses, should they just stop using them even if they have been doing so legally and unhindered for a considerable number of years?

Restricting the use of titles to those who have met the relevant requirements for entry to the particular profession means that titles are used as a form of control by the profession. If you do not meet the profession's entry requirements, you cannot call yourselves X.

Entrusting the protection of titles to the regulatory bodies means that they are used as a way of protecting the public from those individuals who have no legitimate reason to use them. Thereby providing reassurance to the public about those who hold the title and that they can trust those individuals who use the title to be part of the relevant profession with all that entails.

The current mechanism for restricting the use of titles is that it is only after a period of pre-registration education (whether that be in this country or from another country where the educational programme meets the criteria for entry to the profession in that country and certain stipulated equivalency criteria in this country) can someone apply for entry to the profession (via the regulatory body) and it is only on acceptance of the application is the title bestowed. Therefore, pre-registration education (see **Why is pre-registration education a professional issue?**) and the use of titles as a mechanism for controlling entry to the profession fit together very well (you would think it was designed that way!).

SUMMARY

- A profession is an occupational group that has met specific criteria which allows it to have influence over the way it is perceived and its role in society.
- The notions of what makes a profession different from an occupational group has changed over time.

- Various approaches have been proposed to determine what a profession is and what occupations have achieved the status of being a profession. These include the trait and functionalist approach as well as the concept of the profession as a form of social closure.
- Being a profession provides benefits for society, the profession and the professional.
- Being a professional means adopting a professional behaviour and accepting a professional mandate from society. This includes a commitment to acquire and maintain the necessary knowledge, skills and abilities to provide their area of expertise to society.
- A healthcare professional is someone who works with or for patients after achieving a recognised qualification to practise in a specific healthcare field, has current registration with one of the healthcare regulatory bodies, is competent to undertake their area of practice, has a degree of accountability, by virtue of their registration, to their practice and also has a degree of autonomy or independence in how their perform their practice.
- Morals are the internal principles that a person uses to guide them in making choices in their life.
- Ethics are a system for understanding human behaviour and provide a formalised basis for action in a given situation.
- Morals are beliefs at the level of the individual, whereas ethics are a belief system that operates at a collective or society level.
- Shared professional values are therefore a vital element of professionalism and being a professional means aligning oneself to the values of that profession.
- Rather than being distinct from each other, ethical theory and values can be seen to be interwoven in the concept of professional values.
- Morals, ethics and values are interrelated in an individual's behaviour and professional values set out the basis for decision-making and standard of behaviour that is expected of a professional.
- The four ethical principles that are relevant to healthcare practice are autonomy, beneficence, non-maleficence and justice.
- A professional issue is an issue that affects the professional values of the profession.
- Different professions, even within healthcare, have different professional issues.
- Pre-registration education is a way of maintaining the profession's status and in ensuring the professional values of the profession, as well as preparing future members of the profession for their future roles. As such it is a key professional issue for professions.
- Restricting the use of titles to those who have met the relevant requirements for entry to the particular profession means that those who use the services of the profession can be assured of the person's professional status and that they have undertaken the relevant education to meet the required standard for entry to the profession.

REFERENCES

Beaty, L. (2000) 'Becoming a professional teacher' Chapter 3, in Hall, L. and Marsh, K. (eds) *Professionalism, Policies and Values*. Greenwich University Press: Greenwich.

Beauchamp, T. and Childress, J. (2013) *Principles of Biomedical Ethics* (7th edition). Oxford University Press: Oxford.

Bush, T. and Cornock, M. (1999) 'What is a profession?', *Unit 1 in Professional Studies Module*. University of Plymouth: Plymouth.

Cornock, M. (2021) *Key Questions in Healthcare Law and Ethics*. SAGE: London.

Cuthbert, S. and Quallington, J. (2017) *Values and Ethics for Care Practice*. Lantern Publishing: Banbury.

Freidson, E. (1994) *Professionalism Reborn: Theory, Prophecy and Policy*. Polity Press: Oxford.

Goode, W. (1960) 'Encroachment, charlatanism and the emerging professions: Psychology, sociology and medicine', *American Sociological Review*, 25: 902–13.

Goodman, B. and Clemow, R. (2010) *Nursing and Collaborative Practice*. Learning Matters: Exeter.

Health and Care Professions Council (2016) *Standards of Conduct, Performance and Ethics*. Health and Care Professions Council: London.

Macdonald, K. (1995) *The Sociology of Professions*. SAGE: London.

Millerson, G. (1964) *The Qualifying Associations: A Study in Professionalisation*. Routledge and Kegan Paul: London.

Montgomery, J. (2003) *Health Care Law* (2nd edition). Oxford University Press: Oxford.

Nursing and Midwifery Council (2018) *The Code*. Nursing and Midwifery Council: London.

Saks, M. (1983) 'Removing the blinkers? A critique of recent contributions to the sociology of professions', *The Sociological Review*, 31(1): 3–21.

Witz, A. (1992) *Professions and Patriarchy*. Routledge: London.

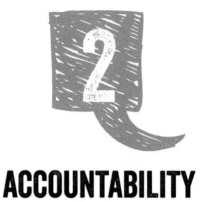

ACCOUNTABILITY

What accountability is, how it is undertaken and how it affects healthcare practitioners is addressed in Chapter 2. This is achieved through questioning the terminology used to discuss accountability, defining key terms, determining who or what healthcare practitioners are accountable to and for what they are accountable. There is also discussion of the accountability of student healthcare practitioners. Chapter 2 then furthers the discussion of accountability by exploring regulation and its purpose and what needs to be regulated in order for regulation to be effective and achieve its purpose. The form that regulation takes is outlined along with who actually undertakes the regulation of healthcare practitioners along with noting how law, ethics and regulation affect the healthcare practitioner.

Chapter 2 concludes with an analysis of the relationship between accountability and regulation through the regulatory bodies and how regulation affects the healthcare practitioner.

QUESTIONS COVERED IN CHAPTER 2

- What is responsibility?
- What is accountability?
- What is liability?
- Is there a hierarchy to responsibility, accountability and liability?
- Why is professional accountability a key concept in professionalism?
- Why are healthcare practitioners professionally accountable?
- Who can hold a healthcare practitioner professionally accountable?
- What is a healthcare practitioner professionally accountable for?
- Are student healthcare practitioners professionally accountable?
- What is regulation?
- How does regulation affect the patient?
- What is being regulated?

- Who regulates healthcare practitioners?
- How does regulation affect the healthcare practitioner?

Q

A

What is responsibility?

Responsibility is a term that is in commonplace use on healthcare. It would be expected that your contract of employment or your university learning agreement/contract will mention your responsibilities in relation to your role and certain things that you are expected to do. However, as is often the case with commonplace terms and words, the term is frequently used without there being common agreement as to how it is being used. Instead, its meaning is left vague.

So before we proceed any further in this chapter, let's set out what is meant by responsibility when it is used in this book.

Often the simplest ways of clarifying and agreeing on how a word or term is to be used is to go to a dictionary definition of the word. For the *Shorter Oxford English Dictionary*, responsibility is defined as '*a charge, trust, or duty, for which one is responsible*' (Stevenson, 2007).

The interesting aspect of this definition is that it links having a charge for which you are responsible. This means that in order to be responsible for something, you need to have some a degree of charge over it. This charge means that you have some authority over the specific role or task for which you are responsible. You can control that role or task, at least to a degree. Without the authority, you cannot be responsible for it because you do not have the ability to make decisions regarding the role to task.

To take two common situations, if you were responsible for a car but had no authority or control over who could use that car, your ability to make decisions regarding that car would be severely limited. Similarly, if you were responsible for the care of a group of patients but had no authority to make any decisions regarding the form of that care or when it occurred, your ability to undertake the care of that groups of patients would be outside of your area of control. Responsibility means to be in charge of something *and* to have some authority/control over it.

A further aspect of responsibility is that it has to be for something specific. It is no use being told that you are responsible for the radiology department without being told specifically what your responsibility entails. Are you responsible for everything in the department? Or the relationship between the department and the rest of the hospital? Or the staff in the department? Or the patients who attend the department? Or any combination of these? Or something else altogether?

Needing to know the specifics of your responsibility is one of the reasons why a contract of employment or your learning agreement with your university will not have as single statement of your responsibility but will instead refer to your responsibilities, and list these.

In keeping with the above discussion of responsibility, when the word responsibility is used on this book, it will be taken to mean: to be responsible for something specific. To have something that is under your authority, that you are responsible for and need to ensure that it is done or that it is protected or looked after, according to the nature of what it is that your responsibility entails. Nothing more and nothing less.

Once you have undertaken the thing for which you are responsible, you have fulfilled your responsibility.

Q What is accountability?

A Accountability is another of those words and concepts that is commonplace in healthcare practice but is often not defined.

Again, it is time to turn to the dictionary and see what that says about accountability so that we can agree what we mean by the term. The *Shorter Oxford English Dictionary* defines accountability as *'liable to be called to account'* (Stevenson, 2007). For the purposes of this book, this means that once you have accountability for something, you could be asked to give an account of that something. For instance, if you had accountability for looking after a specific patient, you could be asked to give an account of how you looked after that patient.

A key feature of accountability is that it is a possibility that you will be asked to give account for that for which you have accountability. It does not mean that you will always have to give an account but only that the possibility exits and is one that you should be prepared for.

In providing your account, you may be required to describe or explain how you undertook that for which you had accountability. Going back to the example of looking after a specific patient, in providing your account when asked to do so, you may be required to describe the care you provided and the reasons why you gave that particular care as opposed to a different form of care. If for some reason you did not provide the care that was required, in providing your account, you may be requested to explain why you did not provide the care expected and the reasoning behind the decision-making that led you not to decide not to provide that care.

Accountability is, therefore, concerned being with answerable for your actions (or lack of action).

Where you have accountability, once you have provided your account you have discharged your accountability for that specific thing.

Q What is liability?

A Although responsibility (see **What is responsibility?**) and accountability (see **What is accountability?**) can be used in a legal context, liability is slightly different to them as it is a concept that has a specific meaning when used legally.

In its legal sense, liability refers to an obligation or duty. In a legal dictionary, liability is defined as *'subject to a disadvantage at law'* (Penner, 2001). This is because when you have a legal obligation, you are legally required to discharge that obligation and failure to do so will mean that you are potentially subject to legal sanction.

The sanction that is applied would depend upon the specifics of the liability, the legal obligation, you have. For instance, we all have a legal liability in relation to speeding while driving a car. The legal obligation upon us is to drive within the speed limit in force at the time and place we are driving. The sanction for failure to fulfil that obligation is a criminal one because the liability is set out within criminal law. It is a criminal offence to speed while driving and, depending upon a number of factors, the legal sanction could be an order banning you from driving for a set period of time and/or a fine and/or a community related sentence and/or custodial sentence.

Whereas if the obligation was in relation to fulfilling your part of a contract, the legal sanction would be based on contract law and, while the sanction can be onerous, they do not have the option of a custodial sentence as a sanction. Most sanctions imposed for a nonfulfilment of a contractual duty involve having to undertake the duty in the contract or paying a financial remedy to the other side involved in the contract.

When the term liability is used in this book, it will mean the situation where you have an obligation to fulfil a duty and there is the possibility of a sanction being applied if you do not fulfil that obligation.

Is there a hierarchy to responsibility, accountability and liability?

The terms 'responsibility' (see **What is responsibility?**), 'accountability' (see **What is accountability?**) and 'liability' (see **What is Liability?**) are often used interchangeably as if they were all synonyms and you will often find one is used where the context actually means that another of the terms is what is being referred to.

As can be seen in the discussion on each of the terms, it is not the case that they are synonymous with each other, and each has a specific meaning that is distinct from the other two. Although there is a relationship between the terms and indeed a hierarchy in how they are related.

If responsibility is taken to mean to be responsible for the undertaking of something specific along with the necessary authority to achieve it. And accountability means that you may be required to give an account of your actions or your non-actions. With liability referring to having an obligation to fulfil a duty with the possibility of a sanction being applied if you do not fulfil that obligation. The nature of the hierarchy starts to become clear.

It may help with clarifying the relationship between the three terms to consider each of the terms in relation to an example. Consider for a moment that you are working in a hospital as a non-medical prescriber and your role for the day is to review the medication that a specific group of patients has been prescribed ensuring that all the prescribed medication is still needed by the individual patients and that there are no contraindications to any of the prescribed medicines.

If you had been given responsibility for this role, you would have the authority to undertake the review and recommend changes to the medication in light of any contraindications you found, or where the medication was no longer required by a certain patient.

Once you have undertaken the review and checked for contraindications and the continuing need for the medicines, your responsibility ends.

If you instead had accountability for the role, you still have the role to undertake and as such need to compete the review and check for contraindications and the continuing need for the medicines. However, at the point that you complete this, unlike when you were only responsible, your accountability means that there is the possibility that you could be called to account for how you have undertaken your role. It is only when you have provided your account, when called to do so, that your accountability ends.

Where you have liability for the role the situation changes again. This time instead of being able to walk away when you have completed the review and checked for contraindications and the continuing need for the medicines (if you had responsibility) or after you had provided your account of the review and the checking (if you had accountability), now there is an element of jeopardy introduced into your role.

There is the possibility of a sanction if you have not competed your review, and there is the possibility of a sanction if the account you give of your role and the review you have undertaken is not thought to have been at an acceptable standard. Thus, for liability, you can not only be held to give an account, but the account you provide has to satisfy those asking for it and if it does not, a sanction could be applied.

From this example, it can be seen that not only is there a relationship between having responsibility, accountability and liability, there is a natural progression between the three resulting in an inherent hierarchy between them.

Q | **Why is professional accountability a key concept in professionalism?**

A | In one sense, professional accountability just refers to the accountability of a professional. However, the use of terms responsibility, accountability and liability within healthcare practice is not straightforward. As was seen in **Is there a hierarchy to responsibility, accountability and liability?** the three terms are often used interchangeably, and this causes confusion as to what is actually being discussed and what a healthcare practitioner is being told about their level of liability. Are they responsible, accountable or actually liable?

This confusion and muddling of terms can even be seen in communication from the professional regulatory bodies (the regulatory bodies are outlined in **Who regulates healthcare practitioners?**). For instance, the current editions of the standards of performance from the Health and Care Professions Council and the Nursing and Midwifery Council include the following statements:

'*As a registrant you are personally responsible for the way you behave*' (Health and Care Professions Council, 2016 at page 4) and '*all of the professions we regulate exercise professional judgement and are accountable for their work*' (Nursing and Midwifery Council, 2018 at page 4). It would appear as if the professional regulators are unable to agree as to which level of the hierarchy (see **Is there a hierarchy to responsibility, accountability and liability?**) they are expecting their registrants to work at. For the Health and Care Professions Council, it is responsibility, while for the Nursing and Midwifery Council, it is accountability. Actually, as we know from our discussion of the hierarchy, it is liability that both are referring to as both refer to being able to discipline their registrants.

It is not just the professional regulators that have this apparent difficulty in the use of the correct terminology. Many commentators on healthcare practitioners and healthcare practice use the terms in different ways and to mean different things.

There has been a recognition in recent years that healthcare practitioners are answerable for their actions because of their professional status. Answerable in this context meaning that they have to answer for their actions and, therefore, could face a sanction for failure to answer satisfactorily. You will see that answerable is directly comparable to liability (see **What is Liability?**) as both have the same process and possible outcome. To see this recognition in action, you only have to look at the titles of article and books that examine the professional nature of the healthcare practitioner and discuss their responsibility, accountability or liability (depending upon the author's preference!). Indeed, the very title of this book you are reading, *Accountability and Professionalism in Nursing and Healthcare*, is an acknowledgement that there is a relationship between the two concepts that have been explored in Chapter 1 and this chapter in some detail and will be further explored in the chapters that follow.

In order to both acknowledge the relationship between professionalism and the level of responsibility, accountability or liability the healthcare practitioner is subject to, there has been a move towards the term 'professional accountability'. Commentators now appear to be using this term to refer to the liability that exists for healthcare practitioners in their professional practice. As examples, in a book published in 2012 examining the standards in several professions, the title is *Professional Accountability in Social Care and Health* (Kline & Preston-Shoot, 2012), and this author used the term in a 2014 paper examining the relationship between responsibility, accountability and liability in healthcare (Cornock, 2014).

Notwithstanding that the Health and Care Professions Council refer to being responsible in their *Standards of conduct, performance and ethics*, where you see the term professional accountability, or even just accountability, you can take it to mean that the author or organisation using it are actually referring to the liability of healthcare practitioners without using that specific term. Professional accountability is now shorthand (even if it is a longer term than liability) for the fact that a healthcare practitioner has a duty to ensure that any task or role they have is undertaken to the appropriate standard, and that they are answerable for the way they perform that task or role and could be subject to a sanction if they have not met the required standard.

It is for this reason, that professional accountability is a form of shorthand for the liability of a healthcare practitioner, that it is a key concept in healthcare professionalism.

Q

Why are healthcare practitioners professionally accountable?

A

The short answer is because they are professionals and as such need uphold the accepted standard and behaviour of their profession. Also, as a professional, they have a mandate with society to provide a service that society needs in exchange for being given professional status and all that entails (see **What is a profession?** and **What does it mean to be a professional?**).

Society ensures that the members of professions maintain their mandate to society and the required standard of performance by ensuring that they are regulated. In this context, regulation refers to the control of an aspect of interaction between the individuals in a particular society and an organisation that provides services to/for that society, for instance, a specific profession (see **What is regulation?** for a detailed discussion of regulation).

Part of the reason that regulation of a profession is needed is because a profession has a specific and unique knowledge and skill set. In any relationship where one party has a unique contribution that the other needs but may not understand, there is the potential for a power imbalance between the parties. Where a power imbalance exists, one party is weakened compared to the other, and this could be detrimental to the weaker party if the stronger party seeks to take advantage of their stronger position.

Regulation in part exists to move the power to a more balanced state by providing protection for the weaker party. This protection is by requiring the professional to answer for their actions and to uphold the required standard of the profession, that is, professional accountability. Where they do not uphold the professional standard, they face the possibility of a sanction.

It could, therefore, be said that healthcare practitioners are professionally accountable because this is a part of the regulation of their profession by society.

A further reason for healthcare practitioners to be professionally accountable is because of the unique nature of the work they undertake and the possible consequences. The possible consequences of poor practice from a healthcare practitioner are fatal, literally. Whereas a professional accountant could lose their client the whole of their life savings through poor practice, poor practice by a healthcare practitioner could result in the loss of their patient's life.

Patient safety is paramount to maintaining public trust in the healthcare professions. Therefore, in addition to patient safety for its own sake, there is a professional self-interest in maintaining patient safety: public confidence in its ability to perform its role.

Establishing the highest standards of service by the healthcare professions is based on patient safety considerations. Brazier and Cave (2016) share this view that it is the possibility of harm to patients and the nature and seriousness of this harm that have resulted in the need for the highest form of standards, and hence regulation, for the healthcare professions. Also, when announcing a package of regulatory reforms for healthcare practitioners, the Department of Health (2004) noted that it was patient protection that was the basis for its actions.

Professional accountability for individual healthcare practitioners arises out of this need for high standards within the healthcare professions in order to protect the public from possible poor practices.

From the above discussion, it can be said that healthcare practitioners are professionally accountable to:

- Ensure that the public have trust in the profession and its members
- Maintain the service by the profession for society's benefit
- Acknowledge the possible power imbalance between healthcare practitioner and patient
- Recognise the possible consequences for patients of poor practice
- Promote good practice through the maintenance of professional standards
- Maintain patient safety
- Ensure that patients are protected from those whose performance is below standard

In answering the question **Why are healthcare practitioners professionally accountable?** it is through professional accountability that healthcare practitioners, as members of a specific profession, are regulated for the benefit of society. Additionally, the profession of whom the healthcare practitioner is a member has a vested interest in ensuring that its members are seen to be competent to undertake their practice, and professional accountability is the means by which this is achieved.

This relationship between the professional status of healthcare practitioners, professional accountability, regulation and patient safety can be seen in a statement from a House of Lords Select Committee: *'the principal purpose of regulation of any healthcare profession is to protect the public from unqualified or inadequately trained practitioners. The effective regulation of a therapy thus allows the public to understand where to look in order to get safe treatment from well-trained practitioners in an environment where their rights are protected. It also underpins the healthcare professions' confidence in a therapy's practitioners and is therefore fundamental in the development of all healthcare professions'* (House of Lords Select Committee on Science and Technology, 2000 at paragraph 5.1). Although the Select Committee was discussing complementary and alternatives therapies in healthcare, their statement applies equally to all healthcare practice and practitioners.

Who can hold a healthcare practitioner professionally accountable?

This question is essentially asking to whom a healthcare practitioner is professionally accountable. Who can require the healthcare practitioner to perform their duty, answer for the way that they perform that duty and apply a sanction if the performance by the healthcare practitioner falls below the required standard?

While there may be several individuals, bodies and organisations who could exercise this power, they can be grouped into a few categories. These being:

- Patients
- Society
- The healthcare practitioner's colleagues
- Employers of healthcare practitioners
- The regulatory bodies that regulate healthcare practitioners
- Healthcare practitioners themselves

Not all of these will be able to exercise their power of holding a healthcare practitioner professionally accountable in the same way or impose the same sanctions, but each has some power and some form of sanction that they can impose.

PATIENTS

A patient can hold you professionally accountable in a myriad of ways, many of which could result in your practice being sanctioned. There are a number of organisations to which a patient may make complaints about your practice. Each of these is a form of professional accountability in that, as part of investigating a complaint, the organisation may require you to provide your account. If your account is not deemed to be sufficient, liability comes into play as the organisation dealing with the patient complaint decides whether or not to sanction your practice.

As well as complaints, patients are able to commence legal action in relation to the care and treatment you provided to them; this would most usually be as an action for negligence (see **What is clinical negligence?**).

SOCIETY

The way that society holds you professionally accountable is through the organisations it establishes to oversee your healthcare practice. In addition, society can hold you to account through both the civil and criminal justice systems. Any action in the civil justice system would normally be through a patient's legal action (see above). If your practice is deemed to fall seriously below an acceptable standard such that this results in the death of a patient, you may find yourself defending your practice in the criminal courts.

Another way that society can hold healthcare practitioners to account is through the media, where errant practitioners can find that they are publicly admonished: a form of 'naming and shaming'.

YOUR COLLEAGUES

Your colleagues can hold you professionally accountable both informally and formally. Informally, they may have a quiet word with you about something that hasn't gone as planned and provide suggestions as to how this can be prevented in the future; the formal route is to report you and your practice through your employer's disciplinary or patient safety processes.

Consequences that can arise are when colleagues refuse to work with you or insist that your practice is supervised.

YOUR EMPLOYER

Your employer has the right to expect you to perform your duties in an acceptable manner, to the required standard and at given times. They will have issued you with a contract of employment, which states what these duties are, will outline the amount of time you are expected to work and possibly the locations where you are required to perform your duties.

If you fail to perform your duties in the way expected by your employer, they can hold you professionally accountable through their disciplinary process. They can hold you liable for your actions by suspending you from your work; placing restrictions on the extent of your practice; requiring you to work under supervision or to undertake further training before you are allowed to practice unsupervised; suspending you from work for a set period or time or, ultimately, dismissing you from the position you hold.

YOUR STATUTORY REGULATORY BODY

The statutory regulatory bodies have defined and published mechanisms in place to hold the healthcare practitioners on their registers professionally accountable. This is one of the key mechanisms by which they protect the public and ensure patient safety (see **What is regulation?** for further discussion on public protection).

YOURSELF

If any of the list surprised you, it was probably seeing that you can hold yourself accountable and liable for your actions as a healthcare practitioner. This is not a legal or formal ethical liability. Yet you should be your greatest critic. It is you who decides upon your level of competence and you who, therefore, ultimately makes the decision on whether you will offer a particular treatment to a particular patient at a particular point in time.

Because of this, you should regularly reflect and review your practice in order that you can learn from both what has gone well, as well as noting areas for improvement. By doing this, you are in effect holding yourself to account. With regard to the liability aspect, if you ever felt that you were not competent to undertake a particular treatment, you should not do so; this is a form of regulating your own practice.

Indeed, it can be said to be the hallmark of the highest level of practice, as it ensures that patients only receive the care and treatment that you feel you are competent to provide.

If you do not hold yourself to account, it is you who has to live with the consequences of your actions.

Q What is a healthcare practitioner professionally accountable for?

A There is no list we can refer to that details what a healthcare practitioner is professionally accountable for. It would be good if there were as it would mean we could simply look up if something was on the list or not. If it wasn't on the list, we could ignore it and not worry about it, whereas if it were on the list, we would need to ensure that we paid attention to it and met whatever it required of us.

It could be said that, although having a list of what a healthcare practitioner is and is not professionally accountable for would make life a lot easier, use of such a list goes against the notion of being a professional who upholds the values and standards of their profession.

A key aspect of being a professional is adopting professional behaviours that are in keeping with the expectation of the profession (see **What does it mean to be a professional?**). If you merely check off your actions against a list, while you may behave in the accepted manner, you are not subscribing to the shared values and beliefs of the profession as to what professional behaviour is. In fact, you could be said not to know what professional behaviour is as you have to keep checking the list!

It is for this reason that there is no prescribed list of what a healthcare practitioner is professionally accountable for. Instead, a healthcare practitioner is professionally accountable for their actions. Not just in relation to the actions they perform in their professional practice but, as we shall see in **Can a healthcare practitioner be investigated for personal as well as professional issues?** also for those actions they take in their personal lives in some instances.

Anything that can be said to have an effect on the healthcare practitioner's practice, or on their upholding of the standards of their profession, they are professionally accountable for.

Q Are student healthcare practitioners professionally accountable?

A Student healthcare practitioners do not meet the criteria of being a professional as they have not yet achieved the conditions necessary for entry to the profession via the professional register (as discussed in **How does registration relate to being a professional?**); although it has to be acknowledged that they are working towards these and as they progress through their studies, they will be closer and closer to meeting those conditions.

If it is agreed that a student healthcare practitioner is not currently a professional, then by definition they cannot be held to be professionally accountable. However, this does not mean that they escape any liability (see **What is liability?**) for their actions at all.

Rather student healthcare practitioners are in a sort of twilight area when it comes to their liability. This is because they are not professionally accountable but still have to uphold the values and standards of the profession to which they are seeking membership, and they have liability to some of the same groups as those healthcare practitioners who have professional accountability (see **Who is a healthcare practitioner professionally accountable to?**), and they have their own unique liability as well.

Patients are able to hold a student healthcare practitioner liable in the same way that they can hold a healthcare practitioner professionally accountable; this is through the complaints system of the healthcare provider and via legal action through the courts.

Society has the same ability to use the court system to hold a student healthcare practitioner liable for their practice, either through the criminal or civil courts. Society can also admonish the student in the same way as the healthcare practitioner through the media and public shaming.

Many student healthcare practitioners will not be working for a healthcare employer while undertaking their studies, though some are supported in their studies by an existing employer, for instance, a healthcare assistant who is being assisted with their pre-registration education to become a registered nurse. This may mean the student healthcare practitioner is a student for two days a week and a healthcare assistant for three days a week. This puts this group of students in an invidious position compared to other students as they have different liabilities at different times.

The regulatory bodies hold no direct liability over student healthcare practitioners; however, they do have the power to refuse registration to those students who have not upheld the values and standards of the regulatory body. This is one of the reasons why student healthcare practitioners need to maintain professional standards and behaviours and align themselves to the professional values of the profession they are seeking to join, even though they are not professionals at that time. Showing professionalism during their training and education is one of the requirements of student healthcare practitioners in order to attain that professional status.

Student healthcare practitioners are able to hold themselves liable for their own actions.

The additional area of liability for the student healthcare practitioner is to their education establishment. Although the regulatory body cannot hold the student directly liable, the educational establishment is approved to provide pre-registration education for prospective registrants of the regulatory body on behalf of the regulatory body. One of the criteria for gaining approval will be to have standards and processes in place that hold the student liable for their actions and practice, including their studies. The student healthcare practitioner will be liable for their actions in clinical areas but also for the way they undertake their studies and the professionalism they bring to those studies. For instance, if the student were found to have plagiarised their assignments, they would be liable to the educational establishment for this.

These standards the educational establishment has in place will be similar to those of the regulatory body they are approved by. The sanctions available to the educational institution will include being able to request the student to repeat part of their studies and to remove the student from their studies. The student could, therefore, be prevented from joining their chosen profession.

Although student healthcare practitioners are not professionally accountable, they are still liable for their actions and, in many ways, this mirrors the professional accountability of their registered colleagues.

What is regulation?

Regulation is a key concept when considering professionalism and accountability in a healthcare context. This is because of the way that regulation relates to ethics and law and to the notion of being a profession.

Regulation does not just exist within the context of healthcare. In fact, within modern society regulation is one of its key features. For Hancher and Moran *'regulation is virtually a defining feature of any system of social organization, for we recognize the existence of a social order by the presence of rules, and by the attempt to enforce those rules'* (1998 at page 148).

The authors are noting that it is through regulation that the rules for an organised system of social order are enforced. However not all commentators on regulation see it as a single entity. Regulation is sometimes said to have more than one aspect to it. These being an economic aspect and a public interest aspect.

The economic aspect of regulation is said by some commentators, such as Ogus (1994), to exist to serve the best interests of the members of society in their role as consumers. Moran and Wood see this form of regulation as *'the activity by which the rules governing the exchange of goods and services are made and implemented'* (1993 at page 17).

Economic regulation protects the consumer from institutions such as manufacturers and suppliers of goods where they would otherwise be able to act to the detriment of the consumer. For instance, Ofcom, the regulator for the communications services, protects consumers for bad or poor practices that the telecommunication industries, among others, may otherwise be able to subject their customers to. Ofcom can insist on certain practices from those industries and organisations they regulate and also protect the actual service they provide so that the postal service is maintained and does not fall below a minimum standard, for instance, the provision of at least one delivery per day.

The public interest aspect of regulation is society's method of ensuring that the members of that society are able to fully interact within society. Allsop and Mulcahy see the need for the public interest aspect of regulation arising because of *'information inequalities between individuals and organizations*' (1996 at page 10). This acknowledges that in relationships between individuals and organisations there can be, and usually is, a power imbalance to the detriment of the individual and regulation exists to improve this relationship in favour of the weaker party, the individual.

It can be seen from both the economic and the public interest aspects of regulation that regulation exists to control some aspect of interaction between members of society and organisations in that society. Indeed, control is a key aspect to regulation. According to the *Shorter Oxford English Dictionary*, to regulate means '*to control, govern or direct by rule or regulations*' and regulation means '*the action or process of regulating a thing or person*' (Stevenson, 2007).

This definition is supported and expanded upon by Baldwin et al. when they state that '*at its simplest, regulation refers to the promulgation of an authoritative set of rules, accompanied by some mechanism, typically a public agency, for monitoring and promoting compliance with these rules*' (1998 at page 3).

Regulation could, therefore, be seen '*as all forms of social control or influence*' (Baldwin & Cave, 1999 at page 2) or even '*as any form of behavioural control*' (Allsop & Mulcahy, 1996 at page 8).

For regulation to be effective in providing protection of the public and economic interests of society and its members, there needs to be an agreement as to what is being protected, that is, what is the public interest and the economic interest of that society. In order to protect something, you need to know what it is you are protecting and also why and what you are protecting it from.

This goes back to the statement at the beginning of this answer that regulation is key to professionalism and accountability. Regulation, in the sense of being a form of control, goes back to the discussion of **What is a profession?** where it was stated that a profession exercises control over the occupation of its members and has control over entry to the profession and over its membership. Regulation is the way in which the profession exercises this control.

Also, at the beginning of this answer, it was stated that regulation is a key concept in professionalism and accountability because of the way that it relates to ethics and law. As the above discussion shows, regulation is a formal mechanism whereby public interest is protected. This protection exists because of legal mechanisms put in place by, and for the benefit of, society. The reason that the public interest is protected is because of the ethical beliefs that exist in that society. Where there is an ethical belief that public interest is of value to that society, to the extent that it is a protected value, a system is established to ensure that protection. For healthcare that system is regulation.

Q How does regulation affect the patient?

A Regulation (discussed in **What is regulation?**) is the mechanism through which patients are protected from those healthcare practitioners whose practice is below the required standard. Therefore, it provides the patient with confidence in the ability of those healthcare practitioners they come into contact with. Confidence that the healthcare practitioners have the required knowledge and skills to undertake their roles safely and effectively for the patient and to assist them with their healthcare needs.

It is also regulation that addresses the possible power imbalance in the patient's relationship with their healthcare practitioners by providing guidance and structure for the healthcare practitioner to work within and removing those who abuse their power from being able to practise.

Q What is being regulated?

A If the aim of regulation of healthcare practitioners is to promote and protect patient safety (see **How does regulation affect the patient?**) and control is the mechanism by which regulation works (see **What is regulation?**), this answer is concerned with what controls have been put in place upon healthcare practitioners with the aim of promoting and protecting patient safety.

A key issue here is how the professionalism of healthcare practitioners and their accountability can be regulated, that is, subject to control of some sort so that patient safety is both promoted and protected. This is something that has been of concern to both society and the healthcare professions.

The issue is not that patient safety should not be protected through regulation but what exactly is it that can be regulated that would provide for patient safety and maintain it. The regulation that is put in place must ensure patient safety, but at the same time not remove the professional status of the healthcare practitioner. Otherwise, the unique contribution of the healthcare practitioner, the very thing that sets them apart from other occupational groups and gives them their professional status, would be undermined which would in itself lead to a lowering of patient safety.

One way of determining what needs to be regulated is to see what happens when patient safety has been compromised and what changes are made as a result.

When patient safety is seen to have been compromised, one mechanism to understand what went wrong is for a public inquiry to be held. A public inquiry is a mechanism whereby a body is set up with a specific remit to investigate an incident or series of incidents whether relating to a specific aspect of service delivery, specific patient or patient group, or to a specific healthcare practitioner or group of healthcare practitioners.

The Inquiries Act 2005 provides that Ministers of State may establish inquiries where: '*(a) particular events have caused, or are capable of causing, public concern, or (b) there is public concern that particular events may have occurred*' (Section 1).

The first NHS inquiry is said to have been set up in 1967 (Powell & Walshe, 2019). Since that time there have been numerous other inquires all examining failures in patient safety.

Obviously, an inquiry happens after patient safety has been compromised; however, one of the features of a public inquiry is to make recommendations to ensure that whatever event resulted in the setting up of the inquiry does not happen again.

Recommendations from some of the key inquiries can be said to have had major regulatory effects as demonstrated by the following:

- *Ely (and other inquiries into scandals in long-stay hospitals in the 1970s) can be credited with helping to drive the closure of those institutions and the reshaping of care for people with learning difficulties and chronic mental illness.*
- *The Bristol inquiry in 2001 led to the creation of the Commission for Health Improvement, and contributed to the development of clinical governance in the NHS.*
- *The Shipman inquiry in 2005 drove fundamental reforms to health professions regulation.*
- *The mid-Staffordshire Hospital inquiries in 2010 and 2013 led to national changes to nurse staffing levels, reforms to hospital inspection, the new legal duty of candour, and reforms to protect whistle-blowers* (Powell & Walshe, 2019).

A distinction needs to be made between what phenomena are being regulated and how they are regulated. Many of the recommendations that arise out of public inquiries do not deal with what to regulate but more with how to regulate something. For instance, in the list above, clinical governance is a method of regulation but does not in itself say what should be regulated. Likewise reforming hospital inspection changes how regulation is undertaken but does not in itself say what is being inspected (regulated), before you can inspect you need to know why you need to inspect and what to inspect.

It is possible to advance general principles of what the regulation of healthcare practitioners need to consider in order to determine what phenomenon should be regulated to promote and protect patient safety.

In a doctoral thesis examining the regulation of healthcare practitioners it was stated that:

> There has to be an agreed safe standard that … [healthcare practitioners] can work to, the minimum standard that they have to achieve in order to be able to provide care to the patient that advances the patient's treatment and progress and not hinder it. This could be established through the setting of rules, for instance through the use of protocols which have to be followed for specific treatment, or through guidelines that allows the HCP to use their clinical judgment provided that they act within the parameters which are considered to reflect safe competent practice, or a combination of the two.

> The public and, specifically, patients are entitled to know that the person who is treating them, the … [healthcare practitioner], has undertaken appropriate training and education that allows them to undertake that treatment competently; whether this be through the establishment of training and education that is directly under the direct control of the regulating body or through the

establishment of competencies for practice, or the establishment of competencies for entering the profession.

There also needs to be a way of ensuring that ... [healthcare practitioners] are kept up-to-date and undertake practice that is contemporary.

There also needs to be some form of control over those ... [healthcare practitioners] who do not comply with the agreed standards or whose practice leads to complaints from those who they treat.

From the above, five elements of regulation are advanced as being key in achieving the primary [objective] of regulation: the protection of the public and patient safety. These five elements are:

protection of titles and registration;

education for initial registration;

clinical competence;

standards for performance; and,

fitness to practise.
Cornock (2008 at pages 42–43)

Each of these five phenomena in the regulation of healthcare practitioners is discussed in **How does regulation affect the healthcare practitioner?** As to who undertakes this regulation of healthcare practitioners on behalf of society, this is examined in **Who regulates healthcare practitioners?**

Who regulates healthcare practitioners?

Before we jump into determining who regulates healthcare practitioners, it would be an opportune time to examine the types of regulation that exist so that we can see where the current regulation of healthcare practitioners sits on the regulation spectrum.

There are several forms of regulation of professions and the professionals that are members of their respective professions. These range from the voluntary regulation that a profession undertakes to ensure that it meets its own standards and values (usually referred to as self-regulation), through regulation that is required by the state and undertaken by the profession or on behalf of the profession (commonly known as state sanctioned regulation), to regulation that is undertaken by the state itself or directly under its administration (known as state administrated regulation).

The main difference between state sanctioned regulation and state adminis-trated regulation is that in the former *'the rules, and the institutions concerned with ... [regulation], exist with the consent and support of the State and ... are operated with the support of State sanctions'* (Moran & Wood, 1993 at page 22). The same authors note that *'the identifying features of ... [State administered regulation] are as follows. Authority to regulate rests on legislation. Regulation may be carried out by a specialized public institution, or by a group of civil ser-vants in a central department of government. The principles of the system are that those who make the rules, and those who implement them, are public servants: they are employees of the State, are subject to the rules of public accountability and their actions can be reviewed and challenged in the courts'* (Moran & Wood, 1993 at page 23).

The three forms of regulation move from the least restrictive on the profession and its members, self-regulation, to the most oppressive on the profession and its members, state administrated regulation.

Ideally a profession would undertake the regulation of all the matters necessary for them to fulfil their role to society. In the case of healthcare professions, this would include the five phenomena that were identified as needing regulating to ensure patient protection in **What is being regulated?**

Grubb has stated that *'self-regulation has often been seen as the hallmark of professional status'* (2004 at page 83). Self-regulation meaning that the profession is able to carry on its functions independently and free of any external influence. Self-regulation is not a new feature of the healthcare professions. Indeed, Allsop stated in 2002 that *'the prototype for self-regulation is based on medicine. In the mid-nineteenth century, medical practitioners obtained the statutory right to regulate their own occupational practice...[this]...gave the profession a large degree of autonomy in determining what the content of medical practice should be, how medical work should be carried out, and protection from ... the State'* (at page 79).

That a profession should be self-regulating to be seen as a profession was noted when discussing **What models and approaches have been used to distinguish a profession from other occupational groups?**

Although medicine has just been held up as the model for self-regulation of professions, as we will shortly see, the bodies that currently regulation healthcare practitioners are not those of the profession themselves. In the United Kingdom, although the same can be said for many countries, the regulation of healthcare practitioners has moved away from voluntary self-regulation.

At present, the form of regulation in place for healthcare practitioners falls between the commonly recognised models of state sanctioned regulation and state administrated regulation. It is a bit of a mishmash because although the regulation is undertaken on behalf of the profession (a feature of state sanctioned regulation) rather than directly by the state (which would be state administrated regulation), the regulation is based on legislation (a feature of state administrated regulation). Indeed, as we will soon see, the bodies that perform the regulatory role for the various healthcare professional groups are all established by legislation specifically for this purpose, which details their functions and powers, and are often referred to as the statutory healthcare regulators. The regulatory bodies receive income from the individuals who are registered with them in the form of a registration fee, although they are also able to receive state funding (a further overlap between state sanctioned and state administered regulation) for specific reasons, such as the costs involved if an additional occupational group were added to their remit. There is also an additional layer of regulation with oversight of the regulators themselves, through the function of the Professional Standards Authority (this body is discussed further in **How does regulation affect the healthcare practitioner?**), which is more of a feature of state administered rather than state sanctioned regulation.

Having noted all this, we can now directly answer the question Who regulates healthcare practitioners? It is the bodies that have been created by statute for the purpose of regulating a specific group of healthcare practitioners: the statutory healthcare regulatory bodies. There are differences between the statutory healthcare regulatory bodies as there are between the healthcare practitioner groups that they regulate; however, there are some common characteristics that they share, and they all share a common function.

The following table lists, alphabetically, the statutory healthcare regulatory bodies for those healthcare professions where practitioners are legally required to be registered in order to perform their professional role.

Each of these statutory regulatory bodies fulfils various requirements for professional status discussed in **What models and approaches have been used to distinguish a profession from other occupational groups?**

Table 2.1   Statutory regulatory bodies and who they regulate

Healthcare practitioners	Statutory regulatory body
Chiropractors	General Chiropractic Council
Dentists and associated practitioners such as dental hygienists and dental nurses	General Dental Council
Doctors	General Medical Council
Optometrists and dispensing opticians	General Optical Council
Osteopaths	General Osteopathic Council
Pharmacists and pharmacy technicians	General Pharmaceutical Council (in Northern Ireland the Pharmaceutical Society of Northern Ireland undertakes this role)
Art therapists, chiropodist/podiatrists, dieticians, paramedics, operating departments practitioners, radiographers, speech and language therapists, etc.	Health and Care Professions Council
Midwives, nurses and nursing associates	Nursing and Midwifery Council

The General Medical Council is the oldest of the statutory regulatory bodies having existed in various forms since its creation by the Medical Act 1858, although its powers are now contained in the Medical Act 1983. Some of the statutory regulatory bodies are relatively new because they have replaced older bodies. The Health and Care Professions Council is one of the newer statutory regulatory bodies having been established in April 2002 by The Health Professions Order 2001 (article 3(1)). Prior to 1 August 2012 the Health and Care Professions Council was known as the Health Professions Council, which had replaced the Council for Professions Supplementary to Medicine that had been created in 1960 under the Professions Supplementary to Medicine Act 1960.

Other statutory regulatory bodies which have replaced previous bodies include the Nursing and Midwifery Council, established in 2002 under The Nursing and Midwifery Order 2001, which replaced the United Kingdom Central Council for Nursing, Midwifery and Health Visiting, established in 1983 under the Nurses, Midwives and Health Visitors Act 1979, and itself replaced the General Nursing Council which had been established in 1921 under the Nurses Registration Act 1919 and was the first national regulatory body for nurses.

Prior to the establishment of the earlier incarnations of the statutory regulatory bodies, rather than there being a national approach to the regulation of healthcare practitioner groups, there was a more regional or local system of regulation. For instance, with regard to medical practitioners, this allowed a register to be kept of those doctors who were considered competent to practice in the specific region or locality. For some nurses, their ability to practise was linked to the hospital they were employed by.

As to how the statutory regulatory bodies undertake their regulatory function, what it is they actually do and how they address the five phenomena noted in **What is being regulated?** as being required for the regulation of healthcare practitioners, this is explored in **How does regulation affect the healthcare practitioner?**

How does regulation affect the healthcare practitioner?

The questions, and answers, in this chapter have considered various aspects of professional accountability and regulation that the healthcare practitioner voluntarily subject themselves to in order to practise their chosen profession. Perhaps for many of these healthcare practitioners, this is the key question that needs answering: how does all of this affect me and my practice?

Let's get a couple of things agreed before we answer that. Professional accountability and regulation exist to provide protection for the public (society) in general and more specifically to promote and maintain patient safety.

Regulation in many senses is a negative and restricting aspect of healthcare practice. It is based on control and rules and adhering to certain behaviours and standards. However, regulation can also be seen as a positive part of healthcare practice. It is an enabling and permissive force. Regulation is the mechanism where the individual who wants to practise within a particular sphere of healthcare can do so if they follow the rules and adhere to the standards and align themselves with the expected behaviours.

Regulation and accountability go hand in hand. In the discussion on **What is regulation?** it was noted that regulation is the mechanism whereby a profession exercises control over the occupation of its members and has control over entry to the profession and over its membership. Professional accountability is the method by which individual members of the profession answer to their profession and to society for their practice.

In **Who regulates healthcare practitioners?** it was stated that it is the statutory regulatory bodies that undertake the regulation of healthcare practitioners and in **What is being regulated?** five phenomena were put forward as the key aspects in the regulation of healthcare practitioners.

What now follows is a discussion of how the statutory regulatory bodies regulate these five phenomena, and how this affects healthcare practitioners individually and collectively.

The statutory regulatory bodies have, as their primary purpose, the protection of the public from healthcare practitioners unfit to practise, for example, bogus, untrained, poorly trained healthcare practitioners or those whose conduct is deemed to fall below that which is acceptable. In order to fulfil their statutory and regulatory role, the statutory regulatory bodies all perform similar functions in relation to their registrants and those who wish to gain entry to their respective registers.

There are five main areas to the role of the statutory regulatory bodies which are concerned with:

- Protecting entry to the register and protection of the associated titles
- Education in relation to initial registration
- Maintenance of clinical competence for those on the register
- Producing and maintaining standards for registrants
- Fitness to practise of those on the register

Taken in combination, these five areas encompass the regulation of healthcare practitioners and have a protective function, designed to protect the public and provide patient safety, an educational function, to provide for the initial education of healthcare practitioners and also their continued education and competence, and a deterrent function, to ensure that healthcare practitioners uphold the required standards of the statutory regulatory body.

Because the statutory regulatory bodies operate through a hybrid system of state sanctioned/state administered regulation, they need to be able to demonstrate how they operate and are themselves held to account. Ultimately their accountability is to the public, but this is through the Privy Council, a body of advisers to the monarch, and to Parliament through the Health Select Committee.

In addition to being held to account through the mechanisms described, the healthcare statutory regulatory bodies are themselves regulated through the

Professional Standards Authority (PSA). The role of the PSA is to oversee the statutory healthcare regulatory bodies by assessing their performance through reviews of their work and producing an annual report on each of them. Where necessary, they can also undertake a special review of a regulatory body or an aspect of their work if this is deemed to be necessary by the Secretary of State for Health and Social Care. For instance, if a statutory regulatory body was failing to deal with fitness to practise cases in a timely manner or a high percentage of the cases they adjudicated were being upheld on appeal. In this way, the PSA ensures that the statutory regulatory bodies are protecting the public and maintaining patient safety in the way that they are designed to. It is important to note that the PSA is an oversight body of the statutory regulatory bodies and does not directly register any healthcare practitioners.

Assessing how the statutory regulatory bodies discharge each of their five main functions will help us assess the effect of each on healthcare practitioners and combined will allow us to determine how regulation affects healthcare practitioners.

PROTECTING ENTRY TO THE REGISTER AND PROTECTION OF THE ASSOCIATED TITLES

The statutory regulatory bodies set the requirements for entry to their respective registers; without being registered a healthcare practitioner is unable to practise in their chosen field. As well as educational requirements, prospective registrants need to meet requirements in relation to their character and their health to gain entry to the register.

The protection of titles is the method by which the statutory regulatory bodies protect the public from individuals who have not met their requirements for registration. This was examined in **Is it important to restrict the use of titles?** where the rationale for protecting titles was explored. Here it will suffice to say that the statutory regulatory bodies control who can use a specific title and can take action against those who fraudulently use them: it is a criminal offence to say that you are registered with a statutory healthcare regulatory body when you are not or to dishonestly use a protected title.

In **Is it important to restrict the use of titles?** it was seen that one of the issues with the protection of titles is the actual titles that are protected. If a title is not protected, anyone can use it which can be confusing and misleading for the public. For instance, 'midwife' is a protected title (Nursing and Midwifery Order 2001, Article 44); 'nurse' is not a protected title, rather 'registered nurse' is. Similarly, 'doctor' is not a protected title, but 'registered medical practitioner' is.

The Health and Care Professions Council (HCPC) has a protected title for each of the professions it regulates by virtue of section 6(2) of The Health Professions Order 2001.

EDUCATION IN RELATION TO INITIAL REGISTRATION

To register with the appropriate statutory regulatory body, you need to fulfil certain criteria, one of which is to have completed a set programme of education with a set number of practice hours and attain stipulated competencies.

It is the statutory regulatory bodies that set these criteria and also authorise educational institutions to provide approved programmes of study leading to registration, and undertake quality assurance checks on these programmes on a periodic basis.

This is explored further in **Why is pre-registration education a professional issue?**

MAINTENANCE OF CLINICAL COMPETENCE FOR THOSE ON THE REGISTER

It used to be that registration with a statutory regulatory body was for life, unless you were sanctioned as a result of a fitness to practise investigation into an aspect of your practice. This is not the case anymore. Healthcare practitioners not only have to pay their periodic fee to maintain their registration, they also have to demonstrate that they are maintaining and developing their competence. This is generally termed 'revalidation' (for a discussion on revalidation see **How is revalidation different to appraisal?**). It is a relatively new requirement, for instance, the General Medical Council introduced revalidation in December 2012 while the Nursing and Midwifery Council introduced it in April 2016.

Part of any revalidation requirement is undertaking continuing professional development (CPD) (continuing professional development is defined and discussed in **What is continuing professional development?**). CPD is a two part process: the first is that the healthcare practitioner has to undertake some form of learning, training or education, either formal or informal, that has relevance to their area of practice. The second part is that this needs to be recorded, and, for some regulatory body requirements, to be reflected upon so that the healthcare practitioner can show what they have learnt from the CPD and how it assists them in their practice.

PRODUCING AND MAINTAINING STANDARDS FOR REGISTRANTS

The statutory regulatory bodies all issue their own standards or codes of conduct, for example, the Nursing and Midwifery Council (2018) 'The Code' and the Health and Care Professions Council (2016) 'Standards of conduct, performance and ethics' (see **What is a code of conduct?** and **Do codes of conduct have legal status?** for a discussion of codes of conduct and their use). They have a basis in ethics and ethical principles and professional values as discussed in **How do morals, ethics and professional values relate to being a professional?** and are designed to assist healthcare practitioners in deciding upon what is appropriate behaviour in any situation. They set out the accepted conduct of a healthcare practitioner registered with the statutory regulatory body.

The legislation that governs the statutory regulatory bodies provides the basis for them to issue these codes of conduct. For instance, the Medical Act 1983 (section 35) states *'the powers of the General Council shall include the power to provide, in such manner as the Council think fit, advice for members of the medical profession on—(a) standards of professional conduct; (b) standards of professional performance; or (c) medical ethics'*; while The Nursing and Midwifery Order 2001, in article 3(2), states, that *'the principal functions of the Council shall be to establish from time to time standards ... conduct and performance for nurses and midwives'*.

Codes of conduct may be likened to a set of regulations for the healthcare practitioner to follow. While deviance from a code of conduct is not itself an unlawful act, it may be seen as evidence of misconduct on the part of a healthcare practitioner, by a court of law or a fitness to practise hearing, if the healthcare practitioner cannot provide a valid reason for their deviance from it.

FITNESS TO PRACTISE OF THOSE ON THE REGISTER

In order to assist the statutory regulatory bodies in their protection of patients and the public, they have the ability to remove healthcare practitioners from their respective registers. This is following an investigation into the healthcare practitioner's fitness to practise (see **What is a fitness to practise investigation?** for further discussion on this).

The statutory regulatory bodies have different, but similar, processes for determining a healthcare practitioner's fitness to practise. For example, the Health and Care Professions Council has a conduct and competence committee that hears complaints of misconduct and a health committee that considers whether a healthcare practitioner's practice may be impaired by a condition or illness.

The sanctions available to a statutory regulatory body, as discussed in **What sanctions can be imposed by a statutory regulatory body?** include the ability to impose the ultimate liability on your practice, that of removing you from the register and thereby preventing you from practising in your chosen profession. Other forms of sanction that the statutory regulatory bodies can impose upon healthcare practitioners include requiring them: to undergo training and education; to receive treatment or care for a condition before returning to practice; to work under the supervision of another registered healthcare practitioner in their field; to be suspended for a period of time or to not work in specific fields of practice or with certain groups of patients.

In conclusion, there are quite a range of ways that the healthcare practitioner can be affected by regulation.

The prospective healthcare practitioner has to meet minimum standards of education in order to apply for registration. Without being registered with the relevant statutory regulatory body, they are not able to practise. Healthcare practitioners are required to pay a fee, usually annually, to maintain their registration. The title that a healthcare practitioner uses may be governed by legislation and restricted to certain groups of healthcare practitioner.

Healthcare practitioners must maintain their clinical competence in the area in which they practise and are required to periodically confirm this.

There is a requirement that healthcare practitioners uphold the standards of the profession in which they are registered. There will be a code of conduct to assist them with these standards.

Those healthcare practitioners who do not uphold the standards of their profession may find themselves subject to a fitness to practise investigation, with the possibility of sanctions against their practice if they are found to have fallen below the required standard.

SUMMARY

- Responsibility means to be responsible for the undertaking of something specific along with the necessary authority to achieve it.
- Accountability means that you may be required to give an account of your actions or your inaction.
- Liability refers to having an obligation to fulfil a duty with the possibility of a sanction being applied if you do not fulfil that obligation.
- There is a hierarchical relationship between having responsibility, account-ability and liability. With responsibility being the least onerous for a healthcare practitioner and liability the most onerous. Accountability being the middle ground between the other two.
- Professional accountability is a key concept in healthcare professionalism because it is the term in use to refer to the fact that a healthcare practitioner has a duty to ensure that any task or role they have is undertaken to the appropriate standard, and that they are answerable for the way they perform that task or role and, could be subject to a sanction if they have not met the required standard.
- Healthcare practitioners are professionally accountable because of their unique position in society and to ensure public trust in them and patient safety by promoting good practice and the maintenance of professional standards and thereby eliminating poor practice.
- Healthcare practitioners are professionally accountable, to a greater or lesser extent, to their patients, wider society, their colleagues, their employer, the regulatory body that they are registered with and to themselves.
- Healthcare practitioners are professionally accountable for their actions, that is, for anything that can be said to have an effect on their practice, or on their upholding of the standards of their profession.
- Although student healthcare practitioners are not professionally accountable, they are still liable for their actions and, in many ways, this mirrors the pro-fessional accountability of their registered colleagues.

- Regulation is a key feature of society and refers to formal mechanisms that exist to protect public interests.
- Regulation is the mechanism that promotes patient safety and addresses any possible power imbalance between the patient and their healthcare practitioners.
- There are five phenomena that are regulated in relation to healthcare practitioners to promote and protect patient safety. These are protection of titles and registration; education for initial registration; clinical competence; standards for performance; and fitness to practise.
- Currently regulation of healthcare practitioners is a combination of state sanctioned and state administered regulation. The regulation of the five phenomena that are required to be regulated to promote and protect patient safety is undertaken by specific statutory regulatory bodies for each of the professional healthcare groups.
- Healthcare practitioners are affected by regulation through the ways that the statutory regulatory bodies undertake their functions in relation to: protecting entry to the register and protection of the associated titles; education for initial registration; the maintenance of clinical competence for those on the register; producing and maintaining standards for registrants; and ensuring the fitness to practise of those on the register.

REFERENCES

Allsop, J. (2002) 'Regulation and the medical profession' chapter 6, in Allsop, J. and Saks, M. (eds) *Regulating the Health Professions*. SAGE: London.

Allsop, J. and Mulcahy, L. (1996) *Regulating Medical Work: Formal and Informal Controls*. Open University Press: Buckingham.

Baldwin, R., Scott, C. and Hood, C. (eds) (1998) *A Reader on Regulation*. Oxford University Press: Oxford.

Baldwin, R. and Cave, M. (1999) *Understanding Regulation*. Oxford University Press: Oxford.

Brazier, M. and Cave, E. (2016) *Medicine, Patients and the Law* (6th edition). Manchester University Press: Manchester.

Cornock, M. (2008) *Regulation and Control of Health Care Professionals*. Unpublished Thesis (PhD): Cardiff Law School, University of Cardiff.

Cornock, M. (2014) 'Legal principles of responsibility and accountability in professional healthcare'. *Orthopaedic and Trauma Times*, 23: 16–18.

Council for Professions Supplementary to Medicine set up under Professions Supplementary to Medicine Act 1960.

Department of Health (2004) Press release 2004/0086 New package of regulation puts patient safety at heart of all health packages 2nd March 2004.

Grubb, A. (2004) *Principles of Medical Law* (2nd edition). Oxford University Press: Oxford.

Hancher, L. and Moran, M. (1998) 'Organizing regulatory space' chapter 3, in Baldwin, R., Scott, C. and Hood, C. (eds) *A Reader on Regulation*. Oxford University Press: Oxford.

Health and Care Professions Council (2016) *Standards of Conduct, Performance and Ethics*. Health and Care Professions Council: London.

House of Lords Select Committee on Science and Technology (2000) *Report on Complementary and Alternative Medicine*. The Stationery Office: London.

Inquiries Act 2005.

Kline, R. and Preston-Shoot, M. (2012) *Professional Accountability in Social Care and Health*. SAGE: London.

Medical Act 1858.

Medical Act 1983.

Moran, M. and Wood, D. (1993) *States, Regulation and the Medical Profession*. Open University Press: Buckingham.

Nurses Registration Act 1919.

Nurses, Midwives and Health Visitors Act 1979.

Nursing and Midwifery Council (2018) *The Code*. Nursing and Midwifery Council: London.

Ogus, A. (1994) *Regulation: Legal Form & Economic Theory*. Clarendon Press: Oxford.

Penner, J.E. (2001) *Mozley & Whiteley's Law Dictionary* (12th edition). Butterworths: London.

Powell, M. and Walshe, K. (2019) *50 years of NHS inquiries*. The Health Foundation. Available at https://www.health.org.uk/news-and-comment/blogs/50-years-of-nhs-inquiries

Stevenson, A. (ed) (2007) *Shorter Oxford English dictionary* (6th edition). Oxford University Press: Oxford.

The Health Professions Order 2001 (SI 2002/254).

The Nursing and Midwifery Order 2001 (SI 2002/253).

BEING A PROFESSIONAL

What it means to be a professional healthcare practitioner is the focus of Chapter 3, those aspects of practice and accountability that relate to becoming a professional and maintaining professional status. Initially, the chapter considers how someone can attain professional status in healthcare, including registration requirements. It then examines the concept of competence and how this is maintained, and how a healthcare practitioner can update their knowledge and skills, before looking at the ways in which a healthcare practitioner's competence can be assessed and how a healthcare practitioner can prove that they are fit to practise. The chapter then moves to look at the professional standard that all healthcare practitioners must achieve, and how codes of conduct are related to this. The chapter closes by discussing the role of professional organisations.

Although the main focus is from the point of registration, student issues such as academic integrity and whether there should be a transition period between being a student and a registered practitioner are addressed.

QUESTIONS COVERED IN CHAPTER 3

- How does registration relate to being a professional?
- Why do I pay a registration fee?
- Is there a transition period from being a student healthcare practitioner to becoming a registrant?
- How is an indemnity arrangement related to registration?
- What is clinical competence?
- What is the relationship between professional accountability and competence?
- Are standards of proficiency different to competence?
- Once I am registered do I need to maintain my competence?
- How up to date do I need to be?
- What is continuing professional development?

(Continued)

- Does reflective practice maintain and develop competence?
- Is clinical supervision related to competence?
- What is appraisal?
- How is revalidation different to appraisal?
- Why is the professional standard important to a healthcare practitioner?
- What is a code of conduct?
- Do codes of conduct have legal status?
- What constitutes professional conduct?
- Why is academic integrity important to professional accountability?
- What is the association between professional support organisations, accountability and being a professional?

Q

A

How does registration relate to being a professional?

In the context of professions, registration has been discussed at several points in this book, notably in **What is a profession?, What is being regulated?** and **How does regulation affect the healthcare practitioner?** Registration is one of the key features in an occupation achieving recognition as a profession.

Registration for healthcare practitioners means to be on the list of those practitioners who are entitled to use a registered title that is under the protection of one of the statutory healthcare regulatory bodies (see **Who regulates healthcare practitioners?, How does regulation affect the healthcare practitioner?** and **Is it important to restrict the use of titles?** for discussion on the nature of registration and its purpose).

Healthcare practitioners can apply for and attain registration with the relevant statutory healthcare regulatory body after they have completed an approved programme of pre-registration education and training, as discussed in **Why is pre-registration education a professional issue?** and **How does regulation affect the healthcare practitioner?** The completion of a pre-registration programme will not in itself allow the healthcare practitioner to achieve registration. There are also requirements regarding being in good health and having a good character. These are usually achieved through self-declaration and through a reference/statement supplied by the institution proving the pre-registration programme of study.

It is also possible to achieve registration with a statutory healthcare regulatory body if an individual meets the good character and good health requirements, along with successful completion of a programme of study from an overseas institution which is deemed to be equivalent to the education requirements of the relevant United Kingdom statutory healthcare regulatory body.

The various statutory healthcare regulatory bodies maintain their registers in different ways, albeit with the same purpose of having a register of those who are entitled to practise in the area of healthcare that they regulate. For instance, the

General Medical Council maintains a register of those healthcare practitioners who currently hold a license to practise, that is, who are registered medical practitioners (this being the legal title for those entitled to practise as a medical doctor as explained in **Is it important to restrict the use of titles?**). However, it also has further parts to its register, one for those who meet the requirements for specialist registration, and another for those who are able to work as a general practitioner.

Further examples showing the difference in approach between the various statutory healthcare regulatory bodies include the Health and Care Professions Council which maintains a single register of all its registrants regardless of their specific professional grouping, while the Nursing and Midwifery Council until 1 August 2005 had fifteen parts which differentiated whether a registrant was a level one or level two registrant (that is registered or enrolled) and their area of speciality, for instance, a children's nurse or an adult nurse. Currently, the Nursing and Midwifery Council has four parts to its register for nurses, midwives and specialist community public health nurses and, since 12 July 2018, a part for nursing associates.

For healthcare practitioners, registration is the main way in which their practice is regulated. If a healthcare practitioner is not on the register maintained by the relevant statutory healthcare regulatory body, they are not able to practise in that area of speciality at the professional level, that is, where the title is protected. It does not prevent the individual from working at the non-professional level because no register is kept at this level, but it does mean that an individual could not work, for example, as a paramedic or a registered nurse.

As such, registration with a statutory healthcare regulatory body is an indication that the individual has achieved professional status and is working to the requirements of their professional occupation group.

Why do I pay a registration fee?

In short, a registration fee is the annual fee payable by a healthcare practitioner to be able to practise in their chosen area of practice. If a healthcare practitioner does not pay their registration fee, they would lose their registration and at the same time lose their licence to practise their occupation at the professional level.

The healthcare practitioner would still be able to practise in the healthcare arena just not at the professional level, and they would also lose their right to use any protected title (as seen in **How does registration relate to being a professional?**).

Some see the registration fee as a form of occupational tax. However, this is not a useful analogy as the registration fee does not go to the government but instead goes directly to the relevant statutory healthcare regulatory body and is used by them. It may be more accurately stated that the registration fee is the payment a healthcare practitioner pays to be recognised as a professional in their chosen healthcare speciality and for the privilege of using a protected title.

The fees are necessary because, as seen in **Who regulates healthcare practitioners?**, the statutory healthcare regulatory bodies do not receive state funding, except in exceptional circumstances. Therefore, they need to raise money for their operational costs to achieve their purpose of promoting and protecting patient safety as determined in **What is being regulated?** Registration fees are the mechanism by which the statutory healthcare regulatory bodies raise the money they require.

AS AN ASIDE: ANNUAL REPORTS OF THE STATUTORY HEALTHCARE REGULATORY BODIES

If you are interested in seeing how the various statutory healthcare regulatory bodies use the money they raise through registration fees, you can read their annual reports which detail their accounts.

These can be quite interesting reads as they provide detail of the money raised and how it is spent, but also provide detail of challenges they have faced and how they operate, as well as information on their registrants and their plans for the future. For instance, the latest Health and Care Professions Council annual report notes that they were 286,914 registrants on 31 March 2021 with prosthetists and orthotists being the smallest occupational group of the 15 groups regulated with only 1,113 registrants and occupational therapists being the largest occupational group with 41,231 registrants (Health and Care Professions Council, 2021 at page 9).

Total income for the Health and Care Professions Council in 2021 was £27,162,000 (Health and Care Professions Council, 2021 at page 26) raised from 286,914 registrants.

There is a vast difference in the fees that the various statutory healthcare regulatory bodies charge their registrants. Some of the statutory healthcare regulatory bodies charge an annual fee, while others may charge for a two-year period.

The current highest annual charge (for the period covering 2022) is made by the General Chiropractic Council which charges £800 per year. The lowest is charged by the Health and Care Professions Council at £98.12 per year but paid for two years at a time.

There may also be fees charged for initial registration and for issuing certificates of registration or for other administrative purposes such as being restored to the register after a period of not being on the register. These fees also vary between the statutory healthcare regulatory bodies.

Q **Is there a transition period from being a student healthcare practitioner to becoming a registrant?**

A As can be expected, there are different approaches to how the statutory healthcare regulatory bodies approach the transition from being a student healthcare practitioner to becoming a registrant with them.

Three main approaches can be identified. Some of the statutory healthcare regulatory bodies make no distinction between their registrants, and on registering with them, the student healthcare practitioner becomes a full registrant. Others do not have any formal conditions but provide guidance and recommendations for a transition period once the student healthcare practitioner has achieved registration with them. Others have a period of conditional registration.

Two examples will illustrate these latter two approaches to the transition from student to registrant.

The Nursing and Midwifery Council does not have a formal transition period for its new registrants. All registrants are full registrants at the point of registration. However, the Nursing and Midwifery Council does recommend a preceptorship period for new registrants.

The Nursing and Midwifery Council has stated 'that the experience a newly registered nurse, midwife or nursing associate has in the period directly after initial registration is significantly important and can positively influence their journey to becoming a confident professional…the preceptorship period provides the basis for the beginning of a lifelong journey of reflection, and the ability to self-identify continuing professional development needs, as the nurse, midwife and nursing associate embarks on their career and prepares for revalidation' (Nursing and Midwifery Council, 2020 at page 5).

Preceptorship is not obligatory and is not offered by the Nursing and Midwifery Council itself. Rather, it is a period of time when the new registrant receives additional support through a structured programme provided by their first employer. This programme may include working with an experienced nurse (preceptor) who can help them transition to the demands of their new role, protected time for the new registrant to meet with their preceptor to discuss progress and achievement of objectives, meetings between groups of new registrants, formal teaching or developmental sessions.

For the Nursing and Midwifery Council, 'the objectives of preceptorship are to welcome and integrate the newly registered nurse, midwife and nursing associate into the team and place of work, help them grow in confidence, and begin their lifelong journey as an accountable, independent, knowledgeable and skilled practitioner' (Nursing and Midwifery Council, 2020 at page 3).

The General Medical Council provides students who become new registrants with provisional registration. Provisional registration means that the medical practitioner is registered with the General Medical Council and so subject to all the regulation that every registrant would be subject to; however, because they do not have full registration, they cannot take any role that a full registrant could. In effect, it means that they can take a job that acts as a bridge between being a student to being a full registered medical practitioner who can take any job anywhere. The roles and jobs available to those with provisional registration are ones that provide support and guidance and have been approved as providing the necessary training to allow medical practitioners to gain the skills and competencies they need for their future careers.

At the successful end of the period of provisional registration, the medical practitioner is issued with a 'certificate of experience' that allows them to apply for full registration with the General Medical Council.

The General Medical Council limits the period of time that a medical practitioner can be provisionally registered, the norm maximum is three years and 30 days, although this can be extended in certain circumstances (General Medical Council, 2022).

While it has been seen that the Nursing and Midwifery Council uses preceptor-ship and the General Medical Council conditional registration, as an example, the General Optical Council has no transition between student and fully registered professionals.

Q

How is an indemnity arrangement related to registration?

A

Indemnity is defined as '*security or protection against contingent hurt, damage or loss*' by the *Shorter Oxford English Dictionary* (Stevenson, 2007). While an '*indemnity arrangement is one that will indemnify the person who holds it from expenses incurred or suffering a loss*' (Cornock, 2020 at page 6). In the healthcare context, an indemnity arrangement can be likened to having insurance cover in case of an incident during a healthcare practitioner's professional practice.

If an incident were to occur, the indemnity arrangement pays for any legal costs the healthcare practitioner were to incur in defending themselves against a claim, as well as any compensation awarded to the person bringing the claim against the healthcare practitioner.

An indemnity arrangement is an aspect of professional accountability as it is a way of demonstrating that if something were to go wrong within a healthcare practitioner's practice, they have ensured that their patient will receive the appro-priate compensation.

As to why indemnity arrangements are linked to registration, this is because it is a legal requirement that healthcare practitioners have an indemnity arrangement in place in order to register and maintain their registration with a statutory healthcare regulatory body. It is a legal requirement because the laws which govern statutory healthcare regulatory bodies and their functions specifically mention the need for an indemnity arrangement.

For example, article 12A(1) of The Nursing and Midwifery Order 2001 states '*Each practising registrant must have in force in relation to that registrant an indemnity arrangement which provides appropriate cover for practising as such*'. While article 12A(93) defines 'appropriate cover' as '*cover against liabilities that may be incurred in practising as such which is appropriate, having regard to the nature and extent of the risks of practising as such*'. The other statutory healthcare regulatory bodies have similar wording in their legislative provisions. Failure to have or to maintain an indemnity arrangement can result in the registrant being removed from the professional register (The Nursing and Midwifery Order 2001 article 12(A) (8a)) or may be treated as misconduct and referred to a fitness to practise committee (article 12(A) (8b)).

Indemnity arrangements have not always been required, and it was only relatively recently that it was made a part of the registration requirements. The Health and Care Professions Council made it compulsory in April 2014; the General Medical

Council followed in August 2015, with the Nursing and Midwifery Council making it a compulsory requirement for registration in April 2016.

If a healthcare practitioner works solely for the National Health Service, their indemnity arrangement will be provided by their employer. This is through NHS Resolution, formerly the NHS Litigation Authority, which manages a number of indemnity schemes for NHS employees for which the employer pays a fee.

The cover provided through NHS Resolution is a basic indemnity arrangement which satisfies the requirements for registration of the statutory healthcare regulatory bodies. It provides cover for claims of clinical negligence (see **What is clinical negligence?**) made against healthcare practitioners.

Those healthcare practitioners who work outside of the NHS may have their indemnity arrangement provided by their employer, or they may be required to have their own arrangement in place. Those healthcare practitioners who are self-employed will need to make provision for their own indemnity arrangement.

There are various organisations that provide indemnity arrangements, such as professional organisations, trade unions and specific organisations that exist for this purpose. The indemnity arrangements they provide vary, and some provide assistance to the healthcare practitioner beyond the basic arrangement offered for NHS employees. This additional cover may include assistance for disputes with employers, such as grievances the employee may bring against their employer or complaints made against the employee, and even cover for fitness to practise investigations and hearings undertaken by the statutory healthcare regulatory bodies. This additional cover is also available from these organisations to NHS employees for the appropriate fee.

Most healthcare practitioners do not need to take out their own or additional indemnity cover for their NHS work to satisfy the statutory healthcare regulatory bodies registration requirements, unless they have additional work or duties outside of their NHS employment. Because the NHS indemnity arrangement will only provide cover for their NHS work. It is generally only the self-employed and those working outside the NHS who need their own indemnity arrangement in place.

The various statutory healthcare regulatory bodies provide information on indemnity arrangements, and these can be obtained from their respective websites (see Table 3.1 Statutory regulatory body websites).

What is clinical competence?

The issue in determining what clinical competence means is that it is very often left undefined and there seems to be an assumption that everyone knows that it means without the need to define or explain it.

For instance, several of the codes of conduct of the statutory regulatory bodies (see **What is a code of conduct?** for a discussion of codes of conduct) mention competence without defining what they mean by their use of that term in that document. For example, see Good Medical Practice (General Medical Council, 2020), Standards of Conduct, Performance and Ethics (Health and Care Professions Council, 2016) and/or The Code (Nursing and Midwifery Council, 2018).

Table 3.1 Statutory regulatory body websites

Statutory regulatory body	Website
General Chiropractic Council	https://www.gcc-uk.org/
General Dental Council	https://www.gdc-uk.org/
General Medical Council	https://www.gmc-uk.org/
General Optical Council	https://optical.org/
General Osteopathic Council	https://www.osteopathy.org.uk/home/
General Pharmaceutical Council	https://www.pharmacyregulation.org/
Health and Care Professions Council	https://www.hcpc-uk.org/
Nursing and Midwifery Council	https://www.nmc.org.uk/
Pharmaceutical Society of Northern Ireland	https://www.psni.org.uk/

The *Shorter Oxford English Dictionary* defines competence as '*having adequate skill*' and '*being properly qualified*' (Stevenson, 2007). On this definition, at the point of registration with one of the statutory regulatory bodies, the healthcare practitioner would be competent to undertake their professional role. Indeed, as discussed in **How does registration relate to being a professional?** and **Why is pre-registration education a professional issue?** this is one of the reasons for the registration of healthcare practitioners, and why one of the requirements for registration is that the prospective registrant has undertaken an approved pre-registration programme of education and training, to prepare them for their role when registered with a statutory regulatory body.

Helpfully a previous version of the Nursing and Midwifery Council code of conduct allows the definition provided by the *Shorter Oxford English Dictionary* to be applied to a healthcare context, as it did define what was meant by competence. In 2004, the then current version of the Nursing and Midwifery Council code of conduct defined competence as '*possessing the skills and abilities required for lawful, safe and effective professional practice without direct supervision*' (Nursing and Midwifery Council, 2004 at section 6.2).

From these two definitions, it is possible to state that clinical competence is concerned with having skills, abilities and knowledge to undertake a particular role and that this is initially achieved through a period of pre-registration education. Also, that competence refers to healthcare practitioners being able to practise in their own right, that is, without the need to be supervised as, for example, a student or unregistered healthcare practitioner requires.

Q

What is the relationship between professional accountability and competence?

A

Using the definition of competence from **What is clinical competence?**, that competence is related to the healthcare practitioner's ability to be able to perform a specific role, for example nurse or physiotherapist, allows its relationship to a healthcare practitioner's accountability to be explored by noting what a healthcare practitioner's accountability requires of them for their role.

Several commentators have noted that competence is a key aspect of the regulation of healthcare practitioners and is fundamental to patient protection and safety. For Montgomery, '*the relationship between patients and health care professionals is based largely on trust that the latter are competent. Membership of the profession should indicate a level of training and expertise which enables the public to rely on the skill of the practitioner*' (2003 at page 133). While the Kennedy Report goes further to state that '*professionals should be able to do that which they profess they can do. From the patient's point of view, it is shocking to think that this might not be the case. Indeed, the need for healthcare professionals to acquire and maintain appropriate levels of competence is so obvious that it would seem unnecessary to refer to it*' (Kennedy, 2001 at page 323).

The healthcare practitioner is only able to register with the relevant statutory regulatory body because they have demonstrated that they have achieved the necessary competence to do so.

The healthcare practitioner is professionally accountable, based on the discussion of professional accountability in **Why is professional accountability a key concept in professionalism?**, for their competence because, as Montgomery and Kennedy noted above, competence is one of the measures that the statutory regulatory bodies can use to restrict access to their respective professional registers and is a key aspect of ensuring patient safety.

Specifically, the healthcare practitioner who is not currently competent needs to recognise this and, as part of their professional accountability, raise this with the relevant individuals in their organisation to ensure that they do not put patient safety at risk.

This is a vital aspect of professional accountability, and a hallmark of professional practice, so it is worth repeating. Being competent means knowing when to act and when not to act. Professional accountability is a way of ensuring that healthcare practitioners pay due regard to their competence.

Competence is not based on a notion of being 'time served', that once you have X number of years as a healthcare practitioner, you are seen as being competent. It is the ability to apply the knowledge and experience gained to different situations. So that the whole of the healthcare practitioner's ability and knowledge and skills can be used for the benefit each of their patients: different patients with different problems and needs in different circumstances.

The healthcare practitioner who acts outside of their competence is failing the professional standard and is professionally accountable for that.

Are standards of proficiency different to competence?

As discussed in **What is the clinical competence?** competence is concerned with having skills, abilities and knowledge to undertake a particular role.

It was also noted that achieving competence is a requirement for attaining registration with one of the statutory regulatory bodies. Standards of proficiency are not used by all of the statutory regulatory bodies but by those that do they are a measure of the ability, knowledge and skills that need to be demonstrated by a healthcare practitioner in order to attain registration with them.

In this way, there is an overlap between competence and standards of proficiency as both relate to what a healthcare practitioner needs to demonstrate to achieve registration with a statutory regulatory body.

The Health and Care Professions Council and the Nursing and Midwifery Council have both issued standards of proficiency for the professions they regulate. These can be viewed on their respective websites (see **How is an indemnity arrangement related to registration?** for their website addresses). In addition to using these standards of proficiency to assess whether a healthcare practitioner has attained the necessary abilities, knowledge and skills to attain registration, both also state that they use their respective standards of proficiency to assess whether individual registrants registered with them should remain on their respective registers.

For those statutory regulatory bodies that use them, standards of proficiency are the standard by which a healthcare practitioner registered with a statutory regulatory body is judged in terms of their professional role and their professional values and behaviours. Those who are judged to fall below the standard of proficiency can be removed from the professional register.

It was noted above that there is an overlap between standards of proficiency and competence, and this is indeed so as both relate to specific characteristics of a professional healthcare practitioner. The difference between the two is that standards of proficiency relate to the healthcare practitioner and their ability to be registered with a statutory regulatory body. Whereas competence goes beyond mere registration and is concerned with the capability of the healthcare practitioner to perform their role effectively and safely.

In reality, the terms are used interchangeably, and this does not generally pose an issue as both are concerned with the ability, knowledge and skills of a healthcare practitioner.

Q Once I am registered do I need to maintain my competence?

A The simple short answer to this is yes you do. Though this was not always the case.

In the not too distant past, indeed less than 30 years ago, it was possible to just have to demonstrate competence at the point of initial registration. That is that you undertook a period of training and at the end of that training undertook an examination which included assessment of practical skills and on passing these were deemed to be competent for your health care role. There was no need to undertake any form of continuing professional development or to prove your competence further, unless you wanted to take on an additional expanded role. Once you had achieved this initial competence you were set for life. (Cornock, 2016 at page 8)

This is no longer the case and, after achieving the competence needed to register with a statutory regulatory body, a healthcare practitioner has to maintain their competence in order to maintain their registration.

Part of a healthcare practitioner's professional accountability is their commitment to maintaining their competence, throughout their professional career and certainly beyond the point of initial registration. By maintaining their competence, the healthcare practitioner is helping protect the public and patients from incompetent practitioners, that is, those healthcare practitioners whose knowledge or skills are out of date.

The various codes of conduct from the statutory regulatory bodies all have statements or sections that outline the registrant's responsibility to maintain their professional competence. The General Medical Council have a section titled *'develop and maintain your professional performance'* (General Medical Council, 2020), the Health and Care Professions Council have subsection in their code called *'maintain and develop your knowledge and skills'* (Health and Care Professions Council, 2016), while the Nursing and Midwifery Council state that registrants must *'keep your knowledge and skills up to date, taking part in appropriate and regular learning and professional development activities that aim to maintain and develop your competence and improve your performance'* (Nursing and Midwifery Council, 2018 at section 22.3).

It should be noted that the statutory regulatory bodies not only require healthcare practitioners to maintain their competence, but there is an expectation that they will develop and improve their competence.

As to how a healthcare practitioner maintains their competence, this is addressed in the following questions:

- How up to date do I need to be?
- What is continuing professional development?
- Does reflective practice maintain and develop competence?
- Is clinical supervision related to competence?

How up to date do I need to be?

It was discussed in **Once I am registered do I need to maintain my competence?** that the various statutory regulatory bodies require their respective registrants to maintain their competence. Here it can be further stated that all the codes of conduct mentioned there use the phrase 'up to date' when stating the requirement to maintain and develop competence (General Medical Council, 2020 at page 6, Health and Care Professions Council, 2016 at page 7 and the Nursing and Midwifery Council, 2018 at section 22.3).

Unfortunately, there is no indication of what 'up to date' means, or how up to date a healthcare practitioner needs to be.

Obviously, *'it would be the ideal situation if every healthcare practitioner was fully up to date; had read every article relevant to their subject; attended, or had feedback on, every seminar in their field; and was aware of every research finding appropriate to their clinical area'* (Cornock, 2021 at page 56).

Ideal but not feasible and not an expectation of the statutory regulatory bodies. Rather, there is an expectation of reasonableness in the updating a healthcare practitioner undertakes. Reasonableness has two elements to it: what would it be reasonable for the healthcare practitioner to achieve and what would a reasonable healthcare practitioner achieve in the same circumstances.

Is it reasonable to expect that you have read a research paper that only came out last week? Is it reasonable for you to attend every course that provides updates for your area of clinical practice? Probably neither of these is reasonable. However, it is reasonable to expect that you are aware of major changes and updates in your area of specialism.

Q | What is continuing professional development?

A | There are a variety of terms used by the statutory regulatory bodies to encompass the need for healthcare practitioners to engage with learning throughout their professional careers. Some of these terms are profession specific, while others go in and out of favour, continuing professional development seems to be both current and commonplace and so is used here.

For Peck et al. continuing professional development is *'the process by which health professionals keep updated to meet the needs of their patients, the health service, and their own professional development. It includes the continuous acquisition of new knowledge, skills, and attitudes to enable competent practice'* (2000 at page 432).

Continuing professional development is related to the fact that the attainment of competence does not end at the time of initial registration with a statutory regulatory body but that it must be maintained throughout the healthcare practitioner's professional career. It is continuing professional development that meets the requirements of the statutory regulatory bodies for the maintenance and development of a healthcare practitioner's competence (as stated in **Once I am registered do I need to maintain my competence?**). It is learning and education that goes beyond the requirement for initial registration.

There is no requirement that healthcare practitioners undertake a specific type of activity to fulfil their continuing professional development requirement. Instead, many type of activities will fulfil the requirement. The key aspect of continuing professional development is that the healthcare practitioner is either maintaining or developing their competence in their area of practice. It is a systematic approach to career-based lifelong learning. Continuing professional development can include activities such as:

- Article reading
- Conference attendance
- Conference presentations and the associated preparation
- Discussion with colleagues, for example abut clinical techniques
- Formal training courses
- Informal training
- Practice reflection
- Programmes of study leading to new qualifications
- Research
- Study days or individual sessions

As well as meeting the requirements of the statutory regulatory body requirement for maintaining competence, continuing professional development can also be utilised to acquire new skills and to prepare for new roles.

It is useful for healthcare practitioners to make and update a log of their CPD activities and achievements, which can be referred to for appraisal and revalidation purposes.

Continuing professional development can be summarised as the way that healthcare practitioners keep their skills, knowledge and abilities up to date and continue to learn about their area of practice throughout their professional career. It assists healthcare practitioners with their professional accountability in relation to maintaining their competence as noted when discussing **Once I am registered do I need to maintain my competence?**

It is worth noting that '*there are two aspects to continual professional develop-ment, the first is actually undertaking some form of formal or informal education training or learning. The second is the recording of that experience*' (Cornock, 2016 at page 9).

Does reflective practice maintain and develop competence?

Reflective practice is a way of learning from experience by actively reflecting (thinking) about the experience to determine what happened, what your role was in the experience, what went right, what did not go as expected and what could be changed for the future. In some ways it is a way of learning through experience but where the experience is reviewed and considered rather than just having taken place.

There is no single way of undertaking reflective practice as each person will have a different way of approaching their own reflection, and what may work for one person may not work for another.

Reflective practice is not a form of goal setting. That is, the aim is not to find an answer to a specific problem but rather to engage in a continuous way of reflecting or observing your own practice to determine where practice is going well and where change could be beneficial.

There are two main forms of reflection according to Schön (1991). These are reflection in action and reflection on action. Reflection in action is also described as reflection or thinking while doing. For a healthcare practitioner, an example of reflection in action would be when they reflect upon how their interaction with a patient is affecting the patient's ability to make a treatment decision. The healthcare practitioner may reflect that their interaction needs to be less, or more, direct to accommodate the patient's needs and circumstances.

Whereas reflection on action is when reflection or thinking takes place after the event has happened. In the example above, the healthcare practitioner my reflect that, although their approach is generally effective, there are patients for whom a different approach and style of communication is needed, and then further reflect on what these approaches may be and who they would be most effective with.

The common element in the two approaches is that the healthcare practitioner considers their own practice so that they can maintain or improve it in the future. Through reflective practice, the healthcare practitioner not only considers a specific experience but is able to understand their role in that experience and, over time, will develop a greater insight into their practice and their attitude and approach to their practice. This allows the healthcare practitioner to change, adapt and improve their practice according to their reflections.

Reflective practice does not have to be an individual event and can be undertaken with a colleague or as a group activity. Though whether an individual activity or with a colleague or as part of a group, it must be a method that the healthcare practitioner is comfortable with otherwise they will be unlikely to gain from the reflection.

Competence is maintained and developed through the insights into their practice that the healthcare practitioner gains from the reflections they undertake and the actions they take as a result of these insights.

Q **Is clinical supervision related to competence?**

A Clinical supervision is not a new phenomenon and has been a statutory requirement for midwives since the Midwives Act 1902 (although the current authority arises under The Nursing and Midwifery Order 2001 (SI 2002/253), particularly articles 41–43).

Butterworth et al. describe clinical supervision as '*an exchange between practising professionals to enable the development of professional skills*' (1998 at page 12). It is a formal arrangement where a healthcare practitioner meets with another more experienced healthcare practitioner with the purpose of developing the practice of the first healthcare practitioner. The role of the supervisor is to act as a coach or mentor to the healthcare practitioner to assist them with their practice. The supervision can be one to one or occur in groups.

For Midwives clinical supervision, being statutory in origin is more formalised, and the supervisor is appointed by a Local Supervising Authority after undergoing specific training for the role. A midwifery supervisor will usually be responsible for a group of midwives and must meet each midwife at least annually, although a midwife may request to meet their supervisor at any time for their assistance or advice or guidance. The supervisor's role encompasses two duties, one to the pregnant woman and the other to the midwife. As such, the supervisor is able to monitor the midwife's practice and investigate any allegations against the midwife and even suspend the midwife from practice.

Moving away for midwives, Butterworth and Faugier note that clinical supervision 'should not be confused with simple managerial oversight ... [and] ... its purpose is to facilitate reflective practice and push toward a patient-centred focus' (1994 at page 1). The role of clinical supervision, although encompassing many aspects of midwifery supervision, does not usually have the oversight function or the ability of the supervisor to investigate or suspend the healthcare practitioner.

Various approaches to clinical supervision exist but most involve training for the supervisors, include meetings between the supervisor and the healthcare practitioner being supervised, with these meetings taking place in the workplace, and the supervision is centred around the healthcare practitioner's practice with the aim of developing their competence through attaining new knowledge or skills. Some clinical supervision also involves the supervisor having a more pastoral role in supporting the healthcare practitioner's wellbeing.

In some ways, clinical supervision can be likened to preceptorship (as discussed in **is there a transition period from being a student healthcare practitioner to becoming a registrant?**) for healthcare practitioners who are more experienced.

Although midwives are the only group of healthcare practitioners who are statutorily required to have clinical supervision, it has been long recognised that it is a mechanism of patient protection, and it has been suggested that 'the exploration of the concept of clinical supervision of practitioners other than midwives, should be further developed so that it is integral throughout the line of practice' (Department of Health, 1993 at page 10). Despite this, to date, it is only midwives who are statutorily required to have clinical supervision.

Clinical supervision allows the healthcare practitioner to maintain and develop their competence via a formal arrangement that allows them to receive support in relation to practice and professional issues from a more experienced healthcare practitioner.

Q What is appraisal?

A Interestingly, one of the definitions of appraisal in the *Shorter Oxford English Dictionary* is '*able to be valued or assessed*' (Stevenson, 2007). In some ways, this accurately sums up the purpose of an appraisal as it suggests that what is being appraised is being assessed on its value to the appraiser. For the healthcare practitioner, appraisal is an assessment of their competence to perform their role.

The more usual definition of appraisal provides the detail on the what as well as the how, with appraisal being a *'regular formal review of an individual's work performance, an interview or meeting with this purpose or to establish objectives'* (Stevenson, 2007).

Healthcare practitioners are generally required to have an annual appraisal. However, an employer's appraisal process may require that more than one meeting takes place during the year. These meetings will be structured around a process of initially setting objectives, checking on the progress of the objectives throughout the year, with an end of year assessment of how the healthcare practitioner has achieved the agreed objectives. The process then repeats itself for the next annual cycle.

Conlon sees appraisal as being a *'structured process of facilitated self reflection'* (2003 at page 389). As reflection was seen as being one method of maintaining and developing competence (see **Does reflective practice maintain and develop competence?**), having a formal process whereby the reflection is facilitated through a structure that requires time to be set aside for it and links it to objectives that are useful for the healthcare practitioner, their practice and their development moves appraisal from being a management checking process to one that is effective and useful for the organisation and the healthcare practitioner.

Gatrell and White (2001) have stated that appraisal has three purposes in a healthcare context. These are: as a developmental tool where the healthcare practitioner's needs can be identified and a means of attaining them be planned (though the setting of mutually agreed objectives); an annual assessment of performance by which the healthcare practitioner can faithfully judge their performance and be appraised of how others assess their performance; and as a management tool by which the healthcare practitioner can be assessed against their job description and any organisational objectives.

It should be noted that the first two of Gatrell and White's purposes are based around the needs and abilities of the healthcare practitioner, and it is only the third purpose that is employer focused, in that it meets the needs of the organisation. However, it should be acknowledged that all healthcare organisations should see the development of their healthcare practitioners as an organisational need.

The setting of objectives for the healthcare practitioner's needs is key to an effective appraisal. If the outcome of an appraisal cycle is a set of objectives that the healthcare practitioner does not engage with, the appraisal will not be effective and the objectives unlikely to be achieved.

For many individuals, appraisal is just a compulsory set of meetings to check on their performance, a list of objectives to achieve, and not something that they are engaged with. However, it does not have to be like this, and healthcare practitioners should see their appraisal as part of their professional accountability. Appraisal can be a mechanism by which the healthcare practitioner can reflect upon their practice over a defined period, and put in place any developmental needs to maintain the standard of their practice, thereby maintaining patient safety and meeting the demands of professional accountability as defined in **Why are healthcare practitioners professionally accountable?**

Appraisals can also be used by both the healthcare practitioner and the employing organisation to move beyond current needs to incorporate developmental needs for the healthcare practitioner's career goals and aspirations, and to set objectives for the healthcare practitioner to gain knowledge and skills outside of the demands of their current role. In this way, the healthcare practitioner develops, and the organisation meets future staffing needs.

How is revalidation different to appraisal?

It was said in **How does regulation affect the healthcare practitioner?** that it was the case in the past that registration with a statutory regulatory body was for life, unless the healthcare practitioner was removed from the professional register as a result of a fitness to practise proceedings. There was certainly no requirement for the healthcare practitioner to prove their competence to practise on a regular basis.

This is not the case anymore with the arrival of revalidation to the healthcare professions.

If, as discussed in **What is appraisal?**, appraisal is about the healthcare practitioner and a reflection on their practice and setting objectives to meet their developmental needs and also about how well they are undertaking their role, then revalidation is a system that goes beyond the individual's needs to consider how a healthcare practitioner can show that they are fit to practise in their chosen area of practice. It is about the healthcare practitioner demonstrating that they are up to date in their practice and that their competence has been maintained, that the public trust in them is still justified.

Revalidation is not a new concept, and the General Medical Council was considering introducing it as far back as 1998. However, it was the healthcare scandals in the 1990s, such as that involving children's heart surgery at the Bristol Royal Infirmary and those involving Harold Shipman and Rodney Ledward, that led to calls for reform which in turn led to government consultations on the regulation of healthcare practitioners (Department of Health 2006a, 2006b) that ultimately led to a government White Paper. It was this White Paper that set out proposals to reform the regulation of healthcare practitioners including the introduction of revalidation (Secretary of State for Health, 2007).

Revalidation is administered by the statutory regulatory bodies. At present only the General Medical Council, the General Pharmaceutical Council and the Nursing and Midwifery Council have revalidation requirements for their respective registrants.

The General Medical Council was the first to introduce revalidation in December 2012, having initially been set to commence in March 2005, the Nursing and Midwifery Council was next in April 2016, with the General Pharmaceutical Council introducing revalidation in March 2018. It is to be expected that the other statutory regulatory bodies will introduce revalidation for their registrants, as the

2007 White Paper '*sets out new proposals to ensure that all the statutorily regulated health professions have in place arrangements for the revalidation of their professional registration through which they can periodically demonstrate their continued fitness to practise*' (Secretary of State for Health, 2007 at page 6).

Although the purpose is the same, each of the statutory regulatory bodies administers revalidation in a different way. The General Medical Council has a five year process while the General Pharmaceutical Council and the Nursing and Midwifery Council have three-year processes.

As an example of revalidation requirements, the Nursing and Midwifery Council requires a registrant to have achieved the following:

- 450 practice hours
- 35 hours of CPD including 20 hours of participatory learning
- Five pieces of practice-related feedback
- Five written reflective accounts
- Reflective discussion
- Health and character declaration
- Professional indemnity arrangement
- Confirmation (a signed declaration of meeting the revalidation requirements) (Nursing and Midwifery Council, 2021)

Revalidation is the pinnacle of professional accountability as it is the mechanism by which a healthcare practitioner demonstrates that they are competent to continue to practise effectively and safely. It is a continuing process with a formal review every three or five years depending upon the statutory regulatory body. Failure to either engage with the revalidation process or to meet its requirements can result in the removal of the healthcare practitioner from the relevant professional register.

Q

Why is the professional standard important to a healthcare practitioner?

A

In various questions within Part 1 of this book, the importance of a professional standard has been raised and discussed. Part of the reason for the importance of the existence of a professional standard in healthcare is, as noted in **Does it matter if an occupation is a profession or not?**, that it is one of privileges granted to professions. Only professions are given permission to set their own standards for entry and for continued membership of the profession, the professional standard.

The professional standard reflects the values that are held by a particular profession. Professional values are a way of setting out the behaviours expected by a member of that profession as noted in **Do professional values differ from ethics?** It is against the professional standard that the healthcare practitioner can be measured to determine if they have upheld the profession's values.

As discussed in **How do morals, ethics and professional values relate to being a professional?**, those healthcare practitioners who do not adhere to their profession's

standard are acting outside of the profession's norm for behaviour and not practising according to the profession's values. It may even be said that those healthcare
practitioners who act outside of their professional standard may be said to be acting
unprofessionally and failing to uphold the status of the profession within society and
putting its professional status in jeopardy, as well as possibly risking harm to their
patients. This puts the healthcare practitioner at risk of censure by, or even expulsion from, their profession.

There is then a need for healthcare practitioners to work to the agreed standard as
part of their professional accountability, as noted in **Is there a hierarchy to responsibility, accountability and liability?** Indeed, the need for a standard for professionals
to work to is one of the reasons for having professional accountably in the first place,
as noted in **Why are healthcare practitioners professionally accountable?**

One possible problem with requiring healthcare practitioners to work to a professional standard is how does the individual healthcare practitioner know what that
professional standard that they must work to and achieve is?

In **What is being regulated?** it was stated that standards for performance were one
of five elements of regulation that need to be achieved for public protection and
patient safety to be achieved; while in **How does regulation affect the healthcare
practitioner?** it was stated that producing and maintaining standards for registrants
is one of the roles that the statutory regulatory bodies undertake on behalf of society
as part of their regulatory role.

Each of the individual statutory regulatory bodies set its own standard for their
registrants, although there is considerable commonality between the standards as to
what is expected of each of the healthcare professions and in what they contain. This is
only to be expected as each of the healthcare professions is working towards the same
goal of providing a service to individual patients and, therefore, the public as a whole.

The professional standard is provided to registrants by their statutory regulatory body
through the code of conduct that they issue (Codes of conduct are discussed further in
What is a code of conduct?). The code of conduct is an expression of the profession's
values as set by the statutory regulatory body that represents that profession.

A code of conduct can be said to have three main purposes. Firstly, it sets the
professional standard for registrants and acts as a guide for their practice. Secondly,
it allows the statutory regulatory body to judge a registrant's performance against
the professional standard. Finally, it communicates the professional values of the
profession, that is, being regulated by the statutory regulatory body, to those who
are external to the profession, thereby allowing them to know what they can expect
from those professionals.

What is a code of conduct?

In **Why is the professional standard important to a healthcare practitioner?**, it was
determined that healthcare practitioners who are members of a profession must
work to an agreed standard, the professional standard, and that this professional

standard is necessary for the status of the profession as well as for fulfilling the profession's duty to protect the public, specifically by maintaining patient safety. Also, that it is the statutory regulatory bodies that set the professional standard for their respective professions as part of their duty to society. The statutory regulatory bodies communicate their professional standard by issuing codes of conduct to their registrants.

Codes of conduct are, therefore, an expression of professional values that allow individual healthcare practitioners to know what standard they should be working to, and the ethical principles and concepts that underpin professional values. This is affirmed by Burnard and Chaman who state that *'many codes claim to be based on ethical principles ... others do not overtly make that claim but nevertheless have ethically based statements within their pages'* (1993 at page 4).

Because they represent the values of a profession at a specific point in time, and indeed of the society they are serving, codes of conduct are not static but evolve. These evolutions can be traced through the new editions of their codes that the statutory regulatory bodies periodically issue to their registrants.

The codes of conduct issued by the healthcare statutory regulatory bodies can be said to have an ethical basis and incorporate the ethical principles of autonomy, beneficence, non-maleficence and justice as discussed in **What ethical principles are relevant to healthcare practice?**

Using nursing as an illustration, the first code of conduct issued for nurses by a statutory regulatory body was in 1983 and was titled 'code of professional conduct for nurses, midwives and health visitors based on ethical concepts' (United Kingdom Central Council for Nursing, Midwifery and Health Visiting, 1983). The latest version was issued in 2015 but updated in October 2018, when the Nursing and Midwifery Council commenced regulation of nursing associates. It is titled 'the Code', with a subtitle of 'professional standards of practice and behaviour for nurses, midwifes and nursing associates' (Nursing and Midwifery Council, 2018).

The title of the current code recognises that the code of conduct represents the professional standard for midwives, nurses and nursing associates. It also clearly states that the professional standard relates not only to the nurse's practice but also their behaviour.

The 1983 version of the nurse's code of conduct was eight pages long, but only three actually contained the code. The code consisted of 12 paragraphs that the nurse needed to adhere to and was preceded by a paragraph which stated that the nurse had to justify their professional standing and maintain public trust in them and serve the interests of the public as well as their patients. There were also three explanatory notes.

The current version of the nurse's code is 24 pages long, of which 18 contain the code. The code has expanded to 25 clauses, but all of these have multiple, up to 10, subclauses.

Reading a code of conduct from 40 years ago and comparing it to its current successor is most likely going to feel as if you are reading two very different codes that, although they share some features and themes, have very different content and underlying philosophy.

AS AN ASIDE: HISTORICAL CODES OF CONDUCT

Reading old codes of conduct can be quite illuminating in terms of understanding the professional values of a profession through time. They can also show how an occupation or profession is viewed by society, and of the values of society. For instance, the issuing of the first code of conduct by a profession may represent when the profession was first elevated from being viewed as an occupation to a profession, or when an occupation is seeking to raise its status to that of a profession.

The purpose of codes of conduct is to provide an overarching framework within which healthcare practitioners can practise. They provide an indication of what acceptable behaviour is. They are not, and do not, provide an answer for every ethical dilemma or problem that the healthcare practitioner encounters. Neither are they rule books to be followed. This has both negative and positive connotations. Negatively it means that the healthcare practitioner needs to interpret the code of conduct for any practice issue or situation they face. Positively it means that the healthcare practitioner has the professional freedom to practise their profession as they wish without having to follow rules, so long as it is within the overall professional standard.

The authority for the statutory regulatory bodies to issue codes of conduct for their registrants arises out of their establishing legislation. For instance, for nurses, the Nursing and Midwifery Council was established by The Nursing and Midwifery Order 2001 which provides that *'the principal functions of the Council shall be to establish from time to time standards of . . . conduct and performance for nurses and midwives'* (article 3(2)).

Although the Nursing and Midwifery Council code of conduct sets out the professional standard that nurses must adhere to, the Nursing and Midwifery Council published supplementary guidance on their website (https://www.nmc.org.uk/) which provides additional guidance for specific groups of nurses, or areas of practice, or for nurses with additional competences beyond those attained at initial registration.

One interesting point about codes of conduct for healthcare practitioners is that the various healthcare statutory regulatory bodies all issue their own codes. There is not a shared code of conduct issued on behalf of all the statutory regulatory bodies, even though the various healthcare professional groups share many of their professional values and standards and the ultimate aim of providing safe and effective patient care. On reading the various codes of conduct for healthcare practitioners, it can be seen that there are more commonalties between them than there are inconsistences, suggesting that a shared code would not be that difficult to produce.

Codes of conduct are not without their issues, and some commentators do not see them as being effective as professional standards as they are written in statements that are too simplistic and general. While others, for instance Stone (2002), believe that they are not effective because, instead of being applicable to the healthcare practitioner's practice, they instead represent an idealised version of healthcare practitioners and what they can achieve, and that this is not attainable.

Q **Do codes of conduct have legal status?**

A Codes of conduct, as described in **What is a code of conduct?**, are not legally binding, that is, they do not have the status of being legislation, and they are not laws that have to be followed with failure to do so resulting in an appearance in a criminal or civil court.

While legal action does not directly result as a consequence of not following a code of conduct, they do have a legal status that relates to their being accepted as the professional standard of practice. This means that, if a healthcare practitioner needed to defend their practice in a court hearing, failure to follow their code of practice could be seen as evidence of failing to meet the required standard for their practice.

Being accepted as the recognised standard of practice also has potential implications for the healthcare practitioner's registration with their statutory regulatory body.

Codes of conduct as standards of practice, as noted in **What is a code of conduct?**, mean that they are indicative of the behaviour that a healthcare practitioner should exhibit in their practice. By not following the principles in the code of practice from their statutory regulatory body, the healthcare practitioner is not adhering to the accepted standard and as such is acting outside of the norm expected. This may result in the healthcare practitioner having their practice investigated through a fitness to practise process (see **What is a fitness to practise investigation?**) to determine if their practice meets the required standard. If the healthcare practitioner's practice is judged to have fallen below the required standard, they face the possibility that they will be removed from the professional register and no longer able to practise.

Q **What constitutes professional conduct?**

A Being a professional is about upholding the values of a profession and meeting its professional standard. In **What is a code of conduct?** it was seen that the statutory regulatory bodies, who are responsible to society for ensuring that the professional standard is maintained, set the professional standard by issuing codes of conduct for their registrants to follow.

The reason behind issuing codes of conduct is to protect the public from poor practice and performance from healthcare practitioners who are not meeting the professional standard. To meet the professional standard, the healthcare practitioner follows the guidance in their code of conduct. It is in this way that the healthcare practitioner registered with one of the statutory regulatory bodies exhibits the conduct expected of them as a member of their profession.

Professional conduct is, therefore, to simply adhere to the standard set by their profession, outlined in the relevant code of conduct. Where the healthcare practitioner does not adhere to their code of conduct, this is known as professional misconduct.

A healthcare practitioner demonstrates professional conduct by their approach to, and actions in, their practice. In this way, professional conduct is the embodiment of the relationship between the purpose of regulation in healthcare, the reason for regulation of healthcare practitioners (as noted in **Why are healthcare practitioners professionally accountable?**), the professional accountability that individual healthcare practitioners have and the actual care that patients receive from those healthcare practitioners.

Having a professional conduct requirement for registration with one of the healthcare statutory regulatory bodies allows the healthcare practitioner to be held to account for their actions in their professional practice.

For healthcare practitioners, ensuring that professional conduct is at the heart of their practice means that they will be adopting the values and standards of their profession, as well as addressing their professional accountability.

A failure by a healthcare practitioner to meet their professional conduct requirements, by not adhering to the code of conduct of their statutory regulatory body, can lead to a fitness to practise investigation by that statutory regulatory body. As a point of interest, fitness to practise processes used to be termed professional conduct processes.

Using professional conduct to adhere to the professional standard as embodied in a code of conduct should not be done just to avoid a fitness to practise investigation. It should be an integral part of the healthcare practitioner's approach to their practice. After all, the professional standard means doing it the professional way even when no-one is looking.

Why is academic integrity important to professional accountability?

To be a registered healthcare practitioner, you will have to compete a pre-registration programme of education and training. When the healthcare practitioner is registered, if they want to develop their area of competence and/or extend their area of practice, it is likely that this will, in part, require them to participate in a formal programme of study.

Academic integrity is used to mean good practice during a course of academic study, essentially being a good, conscientious student while at college or university. A student who acts professionally towards their learning if you will.

An example of lack of academic integrity would be the student who plagiarises the work of another student and submits it as their own. This will not have happened in a clinical setting but in a university setting and so for many appear to be outside of the remit of the statutory regulatory bodies.

It would be wrong to assume this, for two reasons. Firstly, if the student was on a post-registration course, they will be expected to exhibit professional standards and conduct in the maintenance of their competence or the attainment of new competences. Many individuals are surprised to learn that a failure to uphold academic integrity could lead to the statutory regulatory body initiating a fitness to practise investigation against the registrant, even when the alleged incident occurred in their role as a student and not in a clinical practitioner role.

Secondly, students who are undertaking a pre-registration programme of education and training are not subject to the fitness to practise proceedings of a statutory regulatory body. Educational establishments providing programmes of study will be required to have their own fitness to practise proceedings as part of the approval for the programme by the statutory regulatory body. This means that there can still be a fitness to practise investigation for allegation of failure to maintain academic integrity. The result of which could include suspension or removal from the educational establishment or lesser sanctions of resitting assessments or a whole module, or even having to retake a whole programme of study.

Additionally, as part of the approval given to them, educational establishments are required to provide the statutory regulatory bodies with details of students who have had sanctions imposed as a result of an internal fitness to practise investigation. In extreme cases, this could lead to the statutory regulatory body declining to admit the individual to the professional register on the basis of professional misconduct. It is in this way that academic integrity is an aspect of professional accountability.

Q **What is the association between professional support organisations, accountability and being a professional?**

A There are many organisations that provide support to healthcare practitioners in undertaking their professional practice. Unlike the requirement to be registered as a member of a profession through a statutory regulatory body in order to practice as a healthcare professional, membership of the professional support organisations is voluntary.

Some of these support organisations act as a trade union for their members, a trade union being '*an organized association of the workers in a trade, group of trades, or profession for the protection and furtherance of their interests, rights and working conditions*' (Stevenson, 2007). Trade unions use the collective voice of their membership to gain collective benefits for their members. Other professional support organisations are more of a professional support group, while others still combine the role of a trade union and a professional support.

Two examples illustrate the roles of professional support organisations.

The Royal College of Nursing states that it is '*is the world's largest nursing union and professional body... [and that it represents] close to half a million nurses, student nurses, midwives and nursing support workers in the UK and internationally*' (Royal College of Nursing, 2022).

According to its website (available at https://www.rcn.org.uk/) some of the activities that the Royal College of Nursing undertake include:

- Representing nurses' professional interests
- Negotiating pay and terms of conditions
- Providing health and safety representation in workplaces
- Protecting and supporting members regarding employment matters
- Providing free advice to members on legal and employment issues
- Campaigning to influence and develop patient care policy
- Providing advice to parliament and political parties and organisations on healthcare and healthcare policies
- Maintaining a library for their members
- Undertaking research into nursing and patient care
- Assisting members with lifelong learning goals and career development

On the other hand, the College of Paramedics does not have a trade union function but undertakes the professional support functions. 'The College of Paramedics [states it] *is the recognised professional body for all paramedics in the UK, whose role is to promote and develop the paramedic profession across England, Northern Ireland, Scotland and Wales*' (The College of Paramedics, 2022).

The College of Paramedics states on its website that its activities include:

- Advising members
- Providing advice to those considering becoming a paramedic
- Providing learning resources to members for continuing professional development purposes
- Publishing curricula for undergraduate and postgraduate education
- Establishing a career framework for postgraduate practice
- Shaping policy and working with various stakeholders to maintaining patient care standards
- Advising government and other interested parties regarding paramedic practice
- Publishing a journal
- Acting as media representative for paramedic practice
- Providing legal representation to members for Health and Social Care Professions investigations (The College of Paramedics, 2022).

As can be seen, there is considerable overlap between the two organisations and the activities they undertake on behalf of their respective members. Both have an education role and provide advice to their members and act as representatives for their members' area of practice, nursing and paramedicine, acting as a collective voice and promoting their views on healthcare. The main difference between the two being the trade union activities which the Royal College of Nursing undertakes.

As to their role in professionalism and professional accountability, professional support organisations can act as a peer group through which new members of the profession can be socialised into the profession's values and norms. Through their educational and standard setting activities, they promote the ideal accepted view of what a healthcare practitioner should be. Membership may provide healthcare practitioners with an opportunity to undertake continuing professional development and to gain understanding of current thinking on areas of their practice. Although, obviously, all of these opportunities are only available to those who are members of a professional support organisation.

SUMMARY

- Registration with a statutory healthcare regulatory body is an indication that the individual has achieved professional status and is working to the requirements of their professional occupation group.
- Registration fees pay for the operational costs of the healthcare practitioners' statutory healthcare regulatory body. For the individual healthcare practitioner, the registration fee is the payment they pay to be recognised as a professional in their chosen healthcare speciality, for the privilege of using a protected title and to be able to practise in their chosen area of speciality.
- Most statutory healthcare regulatory bodies do not have a formal period of transition from student to full registrant. The General Medical Council is one exception to this and has a period of provisional registration. The Nursing and Midwifery Council is an example of a statutory healthcare regulatory body that recommends a formal non-obligatory period of transition from student to full registrant through a preceptorship programme.
- An indemnity arrangement is a requirement for registration with the statutory healthcare regulatory bodies, and failure to have one in place or to maintaining it may result a fitness to practise investigation or in removal from the register for misconduct.
- Clinical competence is concerned with having skills, abilities and knowledge to undertake a particular role.
- Individual healthcare practitioners are professionally accountable for their own competence and for ensuring that they maintain their competence.
- Standards of proficiency and competence are both concerned with a healthcare practitioner's abilities, knowledge and skills. The difference between the two is that standards of proficiency relate to registration with a statutory regulatory body, and competence is more concerned with the healthcare practitioner's capability to perform their role.
- The achievement of competence is not a single event, but an ongoing process and healthcare practitioners need to maintain their competence throughout their professional practice. It is a requirement of continued registration with a statutory regulatory body that competence is maintained and developed.
- In order to maintain registration with a statutory regulatory body, in addition to maintaining their competence, a healthcare practitioner has to demonstrate that

they are up to date within their area of practice. There is no definition of how up to date a healthcare practitioner needs to be, but there is an expectation that they will be reasonable in their approach to ensuring they are up to date.

- Continuing professional development is a requirement of the statutory regulatory bodies and is the way that healthcare practitioners keep their skills, knowledge and abilities up to date and continue to learn about their area of practice throughout their professional career.

- Reflective practice is a way of learning from experience by actively reflecting (thinking) about the experience. Competence is maintained and developed through the insights into their practice that the healthcare practitioner gains from the reflections they undertake and the actions they take as a result of these insights.

- Clinical supervision allows the healthcare practitioner to maintain and develop their competence via a formal arrangement that allows them to receive support in relation to practice and professional issues from a more experienced healthcare practitioner.

- Appraisal is a process by which a healthcare practitioner can demonstrate their professional accountability and reflect upon their practice, and set objectives to maintain and develop their practice as well as those for their career goals.

- Appraisal is for the benefit of the individual healthcare practitioner and their employing organisation; revalidation is for the benefit of society. At present only the General Medical Council, the General Pharmaceutical Council and the Nursing and Midwifery Council have revalidation requirements for their respective registrants. They administer revalidation in a different way, although for each, it is a formal process by which the healthcare practitioner demonstrates that they are competent to continue to practise safely and effectively.

- Healthcare practitioners must practise to a professional standard that is set by the statutory regulatory body that they are registered with. The statutory regulatory body sets out the professional standard that they expect their registrants to adhere to through a code of conduct that they issue.

- Codes of conduct are issued by the statutory regulatory bodies for their registrants and set the professional standard for their respective professions. They provide an overarching framework within which healthcare practitioners can practise.

- Although codes of conduct are not legally binding, they are indicative of accepted practice and thus are binding on healthcare practitioners, who need to adhere to their principles or face the possibility of being removed from their professional register.

- Professional conduct is the way in which a healthcare practitioner undertakes their practice in accordance with the professional standard of their statutory regulatory body, as outlined in the code of conduct.

- A failure to uphold academic integrity could result in a fitness to practise investigation. Either by the educational establishment for those students on pre-registration programmes of study or by the statutory regulatory body for students on post-registration courses.

- Professional support organisations can act as a support organisation, a trade union or a combination of both for a defined group of professionals. Through their activities, they can assist healthcare practitioners to adapt to their new profession, meet their continuing professional development needs and to keep current with developments in their area of practice.

REFERENCES

Burnard, P. and Chapman, C. (1993) *Professional and Ethical Issues in Nursing: The Code of Professional Conduct* (2nd edition). Scutari Press: London.

Butterworth, C. and Faugier, J. (1994) *Clinical Supervision in Nursing, Midwifery and Heath Visiting: A Briefing Paper*. University of Manchester: Manchester.

Butterworth, T., Faugier, J. and Burnard, P. (1998) *Clinical Supervision and Mentorship in Nursing* (2nd edition). Stanley Thornes: Cheltenham.

College of Paramedics (2022) *About Us*. Available at: https://collegeofparamedics.co.uk/COP/About_us/COP/About_Us/About_us.aspx?hkey=ba7d95b7-53e9-45d0-8645-41002d3cffc1

Conlon, M. (2003) 'Appraisal: The catalyst of personal development', *British Medical Journal*, 327: 389–391.

Cornock, M. (December, 2016) 'Revalidation and you', *Orthopaedic & Trauma Times*, (31): 8–10.

Cornock, M. (August, 2020) 'To indemnify or not', *Orthopaedic & Trauma Times*, (38): 6–11.

Cornock, M. (2021) *Key Questions in Healthcare Law and Ethics*. SAGE: London.

Department of Health (1993) *A Vision for the Future: The Nursing, Midwifery and Health Visiting Contribution to Health and Health Care*. HMSO: London.

Department of Health (2006a) *Good Doctors, Safer Patients: A Report by the Chief Medical Officer*. Department of Health: London.

Department of Health (2006b) *The Regulation of the Non-Medical Healthcare Professions*. Department of Health: London.

Gatrell, J. and White, T. (2001) *Medical Appraisal, Selection and Revalidation – A Professional's Guide to Good Practice*. The Royal Society of Medicine Press: London.

General Medical Council (2020) *Good Medical Practice*. General Medical Council: Manchester.

General Medical Council (2022) *Provisional Registration*. General Medical Council: London. Available at: https://www.gmc-uk.org/registration-and-licensing/join-the-register/provisional-registration

Health and Care Professions Council (2016) *Standards of Conduct, Performance and Ethics*. Health and Care Professions Council: London.

Health and Care Professions Council (2021) *Health and Care professions Council Annual Report and Accounts 2020–21*. Health and Care Professions Council: London.

Kennedy, I. (Chair) (2001) *Learning from Bristol: The Report of the Public Inquiry into Children's Heart Surgery at the Bristol Royal Infirmary 1984–1995 CM 5207(1)*. The Stationery Office: London.

Midwives Act 1902.

Montgomery, J. (2003) *Health Care Law* (2nd edition). Oxford University Press: Oxford.

Nursing and Midwifery Council (2004) *The NMC Code of Professional Conduct: Standards for Conduct, Performance and Ethics.* Nursing and Midwifery Council: London.

Nursing and Midwifery Council (2018) *The Code.* Nursing and Midwifery Council: London.

Nursing and Midwifery Council (2020) *Principles for Preceptorship.* Nursing and Midwifery Council: London.

Nursing and Midwifery Council (2021) *What Is Revalidation?* Nursing and Midwifery Council: London.

Peck, C., McCall, M., McLaren, B. and Rotem, T. (2000) 'Continuing medical education and continuing professional development: International comparisons', *British Medical Journal*, 320: 432–435.

Royal College of Nursing (2022) *What the RCN Does.* Available at: https://www.rcn.org.uk/About-us/What-the-RCN-does

Schön, D. (1991) *The Reflective Practitioner: How Professionals Think in Action.* Ashgate Publishing: Farnham.

Secretary of State for Health (2007) *Trust, Assurance and Safety – The Regulation of Health Professionals in the 21st Century Cm 7013.* Department of Health: London.

Stevenson, A. (ed) (2007) *Shorter Oxford English Dictionary* (6th edition). Oxford University Press: Oxford.

Stone, J. (2002) 'Evaluating the ethical and legal content of professional codes of ethics' chapter 4, in Allsop, J. and Saks, M. (eds) *Regulating the Health Professions.* SAGE: London.

The Nursing and Midwifery Order 2001 (SI 2002/253).

United Kingdom Central Council for Nursing, Midwifery and Health Visiting (1983) *Code of Professional Conduct for Nurses, Midwives and Health Visitors Based on Ethical Concepts.* United Kingdom Central Council for Nursing, Midwifery and Health Visiting: London.

WORKING WITH OTHERS

Healthcare practitioners do not work in isolation; generally, they cannot meet all the patient's need themselves and so are part of a team of different healthcare practitioner professional groups all contributing to the care of a patient. This chapter considers how healthcare practitioners can maintain their own professionalism when working as part of a team, and how teamwork affects professional accountability.

The chapter begins by examining the traditional roles of healthcare practitioners and then how these traditional roles have become blurred and what this has meant for the boundaries between different healthcare practitioner groups. It then moves to look at what the response to this blurring of boundaries has been with the emergence of extended and expanded roles and what restrictions now exist to limit the expansion of healthcare practitioner practice.

Following this, the chapter considers teamworking and raising concerns about colleagues before looking at the ways by which roles and tasks can be passed from one healthcare practitioner to another.

The chapter also includes an examination of the role of those who work in healthcare but have not achieved professional status. It concludes by looking at whether teamwork affects a healthcare practitioner's professional accountability.

QUESTIONS COVERED IN CHAPTER 4

- What were the traditional roles of healthcare practitioners?
- How were traditional roles and boundaries challenged?
- Did healthcare practitioner groups challenge traditional roles and boundaries?
- Do any boundaries still exist to restrict the practice of healthcare practitioners?
- Are there any professional or accountability requirements for healthcare practitioners wishing to expand their practice?

- Why is teamworking a professional issue?
- If I have concerns about a colleague what should I do?
- How can a healthcare practitioner be a professional and accountable leader?
- What is delegation?
- What is referral?
- What is the difference between delegation and referral for healthcare practitioners?
- How are registered and unregistered healthcare practitioners different?
- Is there a difference between mentoring and supervision?
- Does following an order as part of a team affect a healthcare practitioner's professional accountability?

Q What were the traditional roles of healthcare practitioners?

A For many new to healthcare practice, this answer to the above question may seem like a historical lesson. For those not so new to healthcare practice, it will probably seem more like a trip down memory lane. Whether you were there or not, thankfully, as will be seen in **Do any boundaries still exist to restrict the practice of healthcare practitioners?** healthcare practice has moved on.

Doctors and nurses will be the professional groups used as examples to explore the traditional roles of healthcare practitioners.

For all healthcare practitioners, the health of the patient is the focus of their practice. The difference between the professional groups is how they approach this and what they actually do for the patient.

In general, and simplistic terms, there are two main aspects to a patient's treatment, diagnosing and curing the patient's condition/illness and supporting them as they go through the treatment process, although a cure may not always be possible and may include managing a condition so that the patient can live with minimal restrictions on their daily life.

This two-sided approach to patients, cure and care, may be said to have led to the traditional distinction in doctors' and nurses' roles in healthcare. Doctors had the role of diagnosing patient conditions and then implementing the 'cure', while nurses took on the care of the patient during the diagnosis and treatment. The two roles are needed because without one the patient would not have all their needs met. Having both roles participating in a patient's condition results in a more holistic approach to healthcare practice and to an individual patient's healthcare experience.

Patients benefit by having both doctors and nurses involved in their care and treatment.

While the role of the doctor may have been seen as clear cut in that they were the ones who diagnosed the patient and implemented any treatment they needed, the role of the nurse as carer was sometimes seen as a lesser role and one in need of defining and explaining.

In the 1960s, a seminal work on the essence of nursing was published, within which it was proposed that nursing comprised both unique and collaborative roles (Henderson, 1966). The unique element was concerned with those aspects of the patient's healthcare needs that the nurse could initiate and/or control relating to assisting patients with activities they would normally undertake but which their condition and/or treatment leaves them unable to. The collaborative role came into play when nurses interacted with others to meet the patient's healthcare needs, such as with doctors to initiate treatment.

For Henderson, there was interdependency between the nurse and the doctor, and each was dependent on the other to meet the patient's healthcare needs. Clarke (1991) advanced Henderson's notion of the nurse's unique role by suggesting that the nurse's unique role was concerned with empowering patients to take charge of their own healthcare needs and goals. It was seen as strength of the nurse's role that they concentrated on the individual patient rather than on the cure or treatment.

Having seen the traditional roles that doctors and nurses performed it is time to consider the relationship that existed between the two practitioner groups.

In a court case that is over 80 years old, a power relationship between doctors and nurses can be seen to exist. According to the judge in the case, '*it is part of the nurses' duty as servants of the hospital, to attend the surgeons and physicians and carry out their orders*'. He goes on to say, '*I would suppose that the first thing required of a nurse would be an unhesitating obedience to the orders of the surgeon*' (Gold and Others v Essex County Council [1942] at pages 249–250).

The case just discussed predated the introduction of the National Health Service (NHS) but the power relationship between doctors and nurses continued into the NHS. As Field and Taylor note '*the final agreement between the government and the medical profession guaranteed the professional autonomy and clinical freedom of doctors ... the NHS thus confirmed the power of the medical profession, especially the medical hierarchy, over other health professionals, including nurses*' (1997 at page 33).

The House of Lords confirmed, in a legal case brought by the Royal College of Nursing, that it is doctors who have responsibility for treatment of the patient, and the nurse has responsibility for following the instructions of the doctor (Royal College of Nursing of the United Kingdom v Department of Health and Social Security [1981]). Responsibility in this sense is the same as professional responsibility as defined in **Why is professional accountability a key concept in professionalism?**

The above highlights that doctors made decision regarding a patient's diagnosis and treatment, and the nurse's role was to follow the doctor's instructions and provide nursing care as appropriate. This relationship was accepted by nurses as the first international code for nurses confirms. One of the tenets in that code stated that '*the nurse is under the obligation to carry out the physician's orders intelligently and loyally and to refuse to participate in unethical procedures*' (International Council of Nurses, 1953).

As well as being the decision maker, the doctor who had issued the instructions to the nurse was able to hold the nurse accountable.

How were traditional roles and boundaries challenged?

The traditional roles presented in **What were the traditional roles of healthcare practitioners?** do not exist as they did 40 or 30 years ago. The nurse is no longer accountable to the doctor any more than to their other colleagues and have their own professional accountability. Something led to these changes and as will be seen a number of influences led to a blurring of the boundaries between roles that occurred from the 1990s onwards.

The influences on the blurring of roles and boundaries between the various healthcare practitioner groups can arise externally to any of the healthcare professions and outside of their control or from within one or more of them. Here the external influences will be discussed.

Doyal and Cameron note that the need for changes in the traditional roles of healthcare practitioners had been around for some time before it actually happened, stating that *'since the 1970s there have been irresistible pressures towards collaborative working across traditional boundaries'* (2000 at page 1023).

In 1995, Dowling et al. put forward several reasons why the roles of healthcare practitioners and the boundaries between them needed changing. They asserted that *'the boundaries between the clinical work of doctors and that of nurses in the acute sector are being redrawn owing to a complex mixture of pressures coming from new technologies and treatments, changing patterns of health care delivery, and the processes by which services are purchased and provided'* (Dowling et al., 1995 at page 309).

Changes in NHS strategy and reform of healthcare and healthcare provision have arguably led to some of the biggest blurring of roles and boundaries. A look at a number of reforms will illustrate how they have led to role change and blurring of boundaries between healthcare practitioner professional groups.

Making a Difference, the 1999 strategy paper from the Department of Health, was instrumental in increasing the nursing contribution to healthcare practice and in shifting the boundaries within which nurses had traditionally worked. It was stated that *'developing roles and improving services go hand in hand. Using nursing, midwifery and health visiting expertise more effectively as part of multidisciplinary team development is good for patients ... We support and want to encourage these developments. We expect NHS organisations to support the role developments we have proposed and to continue to support, monitor and evaluate those now taking place'* (Department of Health, 1999a at paragraphs 10.46 and 10.47).

Following on from the 1999 strategy, The NHS Plan of 2000 from the Secretary of State for Health saw new roles being advocated for many groups of healthcare practitioner as well as the removal of barriers that were said to be holding back the development of healthcare practice. Indeed, the NHS plan went so far as to state that *'the new approach will shatter the old demarcations which have held back staff and slowed down care. NHS employers will be required to empower appropriately qualified nurses, midwives and therapists to undertake a wider range of clinical tasks including the right to make and receive referrals, admit and discharge patients, order investigations and diagnostic tests, run clinics and prescribe drugs'* (Secretary of State for Health, 2000 at paragraph 9.5).

There was certainly a push for reform of the traditional roles that healthcare practitioners had been tied to and for a removal of the boundaries which had been established to protect those roles and limit any expansion of roles to date.

A position paper released in 2001 by the Department of Health reiterated the government's commitments to changes to the roles of healthcare practitioners and removal of boundaries that stifled role change, as well as providing some of the reasons this was actively being sought. Within the position paper was a section titled 'new ways of working' that contained the following statement: *'over the last few years many doctors, and the clinical teams in which they work, have identified new ways of delivering care which have made their services more responsive to patients, more effective and more efficient ... an ethos of multi-professional team-based practice is becoming the dominant way of delivering services'* (Department of Health, 2001 at page 4).

It has to be acknowledged that as well as the desire to affect change in the way that healthcare was to be delivered in the future, there was an additional reason for wanting to develop new roles for healthcare practitioners and to remove the traditional boundaries that separated the practitioner groups. This was to address the reduction in the working hours of junior doctors.

The working hours of junior doctors were reduced on two fronts. A 1993 report on medical training (Department of Health 1993) had made recommendations that specialist training for junior doctors should be shortened, meaning that there would be an overall reduction in the number of hours available to be provided by junior doctors. Coupled with this was a need to comply with European legislation that limited the number of hours that could be worked in a week. Junior doctors were initially excluded from the legislation, but subsequent amendments to the legislation included them within its scope (The Working Time Regulations 1999). Junior doctors' working hours per week were initially reduced to a maximum of 72 hours and then, from 2009, to 48 hours.

As a result of the policy changes introduced and the reduction in junior doctors' hours, the non-medical healthcare practitioner groups saw an increase in opportunities for a move away for their traditional roles and a blurring of the traditional boundaries that had existed.

Q **Did healthcare practitioner groups challenge traditional roles and boundaries?**

A While **How were traditional roles and boundaries challenged?** discussed influences external to the healthcare practitioner groups that challenged traditional roles and boundaries, there was an impetus to challenge them by the healthcare practitioner groups, individually and collectively, as well.

Nursing will again be used as a case study to explore this aspect of challenging traditional roles and boundaries.

Traditionally, nurses were only able to undertake roles and tasks that they had been taught during their basic training. Anything outside of this was not a role that could be undertaken unless the nurse specifically received permission (Royal College of Nursing and British Medical Association, 1978). It has been said that this led to a task-based mentality for nursing until the changes discussed below began to have an effect on nursing as a whole (Naughton & Nolan, 1998).

The permission to undertake tasks outside of those acquired during basic training was known as an extended role (Department of Health and Social Security, 1977). To be able to undertake extended roles, such as venepuncture or intravenous injections, the nurse had to attend an approved course, be certified as being competent, be authorised to undertake the task by their employer, and then had to practise under the supervision of a doctor who delegated the task to them (for a discussion of delegation and its application in healthcare practice see **What is delegation?** and **What is the difference between delegation and referral for healthcare practitioners?**). This was another way that doctors held nurses accountable (see **What were the traditional roles of healthcare practitioners?** where this was first raised). Although the nurse had been certified as competent to undertake the task, they usually had a protocol to follow whenever they performed that task.

A rather annoying aspect of extended role certification was that it was employer specific. If the nurse moved employer, they had to attend another course and be recertified as competent as employers would usually not accept a certificate from another employer as denoting competence in the task.

In 1992, the then statutory regulatory body for nurses, the United Kingdom Central Council for Nursing, Midwifery and Health Visiting (UKCC), published two documents that pushed hard at the traditional roles and boundaries.

The first was a revised code of conduct that acknowledged that nurses worked in a team but also had a contribution that was all theirs, within the clause that nurses should '*work in a collaborative and cooperative manner with health-care professionals and others involved in providing care, and recognise and respect their particular contributions within the care team*' (United Kingdom Central Council for Nursing, Midwifery and Health Visiting, 1992a at clause 6).

The second document was 'The Scope of Professional Practice' position paper (United Kingdom Central Council for Nursing, Midwifery and Health Visiting, 1992b). This was a ground-breaking document. Its effect on nursing at the time and on the future role of nursing cannot be overstated.

The 'Scope of Professional Practice' ... was a landmark position paper for the development of nursing practice. The UKCC effectively removed the need for nurses, midwives and health visitors to achieve extended training certificates issued on the completion of study days before being able to perform a particular procedure. Instead, the nurse was able to decide, using their professional judgment, whether they had the necessary skills knowledge and ability to undertake any procedure that was necessary for the care of their patients, and to decide what skills and knowledge they needed to develop their practice. Where the nurse was confident of their competence they were able to undertake that procedure, where they were not confident of their competence they were to gain assistance from a professional colleague, nurse or doctor, in performing the procedure, or to request that individual to undertake the procedure for them.

The 'Scope of Professional Practice' position paper provided a framework that encouraged nurses to be flexible in their approach to care delivery and to adapt to the changing health care environment by extending the boundaries of their practice whilst keeping the patient as the focus of their efforts. It encouraged nurses, midwives and health visitors to consider how their practice could meet patient needs; 'whilst' at the same time emphasising that accountability for their practice rested with the individual nurses, midwives and health visitors and that they needed to ensure that their practice was based upon knowledge, skills and competence and that they needed to attain, maintain and develop these. As a result, there has been an abolition of the term extended role, nurses can perform any task, procedure or role, not restricted by legislation, [for those roles that are still legally restricted see **Do any boundaries still exist to restrict the practice of healthcare practitioners?**] that they feel competent to undertake, thus liberating nurses from the previous bureaucratic process of developing roles and resulting in the removing of boundaries to the development of nursing practice (Cornock, 2008 at pages 113–114).

As the UKCC stated, '*it is the Council's principles for practice rather than certificates for tasks which should form the basis for adjustments to the scope of practice*' (United Kingdom Central Council for Nursing, Midwifery and Health Visiting, 1992b at page 8).

Removing the need for a nurse to be certified in an extended role before they could undertake that task was to see major changes in the development of nursing practice. Achieving its aim of expanding the scope of nursing practice, as well as removing boundaries to practice, can be said to have ultimately led to the establishment of roles such as the Nurse Practitioner and Nurse Consultant.

Such was the change that the 'Scope of professional practice' heralded that, five years later, the General Secretary of the Royal College of Nursing stated that '*nurses are continuously pushing at the boundaries of care. We are creating new and expanding roles, based on our skills and experience. As a result, we are raising standards of patient care*' (Royal College of Nursing, 1997 at page 2).

Another three years later and the Chief Nursing Officer outlined, in the NHS Plan, ten key roles that they saw nurse as being able to perform. The ten key roles are: '*to order diagnostic investigations such as pathology tests and x-rays; to admit and receive referrals direct, say, to a therapist or a pain consultant; to admit and discharge patients for specified conditions and within agreed protocols; to manage patient caseloads, say for diabetes or rheumatology; to run clinics, say, for ophthalmology or dermatology; to prescribe medicines and treatments; to carry out a wide range of resuscitation procedures including defibrillation; to perform minor surgery and outpatient procedures; to triage patients using the latest IT to the most appropriate health professional; and, to take the lead in the way health services are organised and in the way that they are run*' (Secretary of State for Health, 2000 at paragraph 9.5).

This was to further blur the boundaries between the various healthcare practitioner groups as these roles were predominately the preserve of doctors.

A modernisation of the pay and conditions of NHS staff, except doctors and dentists, provided further impetus to challenge the traditional roles and boundaries. 'Agenda for Change' (Department of Health (1999b) was influential in this regard because, instead of paying someone for the job title they had, they were instead paid according to the skills and abilities they had. Thus, there was an incentive for healthcare practitioners to extend the scope of their practice by developing their skills and their responsibilities.

The new roles that were being introduced may not seem that impressive now, as they are commonplace and many have been superseded, but at the time they were truly ground-breaking. Such was the impact of the new roles that they were regularly reported in the professional press and noted in press releases from the Department of Health.

A few examples may illustrate the scope of these new roles:

- In 1998, it was reported that Central Middlesex Hospital NHS Trust in London employed a radiographer as a clinical practitioner, '*enhancing her role to incorporate procedures that were previously the domain of junior doctors in pretty much the same way as nurse practitioners are*' (Glover, 1998 at page 37).
- In 1999, it was reported that '*Northwick Park Hospital in London was advertising for paramedics to fill vacancies in an A & E department during the winter months*' (Glover, 1999 at page 31).
- In March 2004, the first pharmacists to qualify as supplementary prescribers were announced (Department of Health, 2004).
- In 2004, it was reported that Physiotherapists would be able to request investigations such as Magnetic Resonance Imaging scans (Laird, 2004).
- In 2005, it was announced that paramedics would see their role being developed to undertake diagnosis, prescribe and be able to refer patients and admit them to specialist services (Department of Health, 2005).

Do any boundaries still exist to restrict the practice of healthcare practitioners?

As has been noted in previous questions in this chapter, many of the boundaries that limited the roles of healthcare practitioners now cease to exist.

For a healthcare practitioner group to be able to expand their scope of practice and move beyond the traditional boundaries, the practitioner group that traditionally performed that area of practice has to relinquish it, or at least agree to share it. Many of the boundaries that have been blurred originally existed around roles undertaken by doctors. **Did healthcare practitioner groups challenge traditional roles and boundaries?** examined some of the reasons why roles traditionally undertaken by doctors had their boundaries removed so that the role was available for other healthcare practitioners to undertake.

It was only relatively recently that many of the roles that are commonplace for the non-medical healthcare practitioner to perform today were the exclusive preserve of doctors. As an illustration, prescribing, which was traditionally only undertaken by doctors and dentists, is a common aspect of the practice of many different healthcare practitioner groups. Prescribing has become so commonplace that the most recent iteration of the Nursing and Midwifery Council's standards for pre-registration nursing programmes, the so-called Future Nurse curriculum that is currently being taught, has a requirement that, on registration with the Nursing and Midwifery Council, the healthcare practitioners graduating from the programmes are ready to complete a qualification in prescribing (Nursing and Midwifery Council, 2018a).

It wasn't always such a ubiquitous role for healthcare practitioners. Despite various recommendations for nurses to be able to prescribe since the mid to late 1980s, such as the Crown Report (Department of Health, 1989), legislation provision was only introduced in 1992 with the enactment of the Medicinal Products: Prescription by Nurses Act 1992. It took until the Health and Social Care Act 2001 for groups other than nurses to be considered for a prescribing role and it was 2003 before the necessary legislation was passed allowing healthcare practitioners other than doctors, dentists and nurses to have prescribing as part of their practice.

As can be seen with the prescribing example just discussed, it can take legislation to be passed before some of the roles within the doctor's remit can be undertaken by other groups of healthcare practitioners. This is because many of the boundaries that existed, and still exist as we will shortly see, arise in law and a law remains in place until it is either repealed (removed from the law of the land) or superseded by later legislation.

Until the introduction of The Social Security (Medical Evidence) and Statutory Sick Pay (Medical Evidence) (Amendment) (No. 2) Regulations 2022 only doctors could certify fit notes, that is, sign people off sick from work. On 1 July 2022, this role could be undertaken by other healthcare practitioners such as nurses, occupational therapists, pharmacists and physiotherapists.

At present the boundaries that exist which restrict certain roles from all healthcare practitioners are relatively few. They are the roles legally restricted to doctors (registered medical practitioner is generally the term used in the legislation):

- The Abortion Act 1967 limits the authorisation and supervision of abortion to doctors.
- Section 1 of the Tattooing of Minors Act 1969 makes it an '*offence to tattoo a person under the age of eighteen except when the tattoo is performed for medical reasons by a duly qualified medical practitioner or by a person working under his direction*'.

- The Births and Deaths Registration Act 1953 only authorises doctors to certify death, although other healthcare practitioners may verify that death has occurred.
- Due to the Female Genital Mutilation Act 2003, only doctors may perform female genital mutilation, unless it is necessary in connection with labour or birth where a midwife may undertake it.

In addition, under the provision of section 45 of The Nursing and Midwifery Order 2001, only doctors and midwives can attend a woman in childbirth. The only exceptions are if there is a need of '*sudden or urgent necessity*' or where a student doctor or midwife attends the woman as part of their training.

Apart from the specific roles which are enshrined in legislation as being the preserve of doctors or doctors and midwives, there are no boundaries on the roles that healthcare practitioners may undertake.

Q Are there any professional or accountability requirements for healthcare practitioners wishing to expand their practice?

A Although the boundaries that resulted in the traditional roles of healthcare practitioners have been removed, as discussed in **Did healthcare practitioner groups challenge traditional roles and boundaries?**, healthcare practitioners cannot just include any role or task in their practice. Restrictions still exist that limit whether a healthcare practitioner can perform a particular role or task. The current restrictions on a healthcare practitioner's practice, other than the legal ones discussed in **Do any boundaries still exist to restrict the practice of healthcare practitioners?**, fall within three interrelated requirements.

These requirements are:

- The healthcare practitioner being competent
- Authority from the healthcare practitioner's employer
- Meeting regulatory obligations

THE HEALTHCARE PRACTITIONER BEING COMPETENT

Competence was discussed in **What is clinical competence?** and the information there will not be repeated here. However, there are some points that need to be made regarding competence in relation to healthcare practitioner's expanding the scope of their practice.

Any healthcare practitioner who wishes to expand their area of practice needs to ensure that they are competent in that role or task before they undertake it without supervision. Competence means having the necessary knowledge skills and abilities to safely undertake a role or task.

Because there is no longer a requirement to obtain a certificate of competence prior to undertaking many roles and tasks that extend practice, the onus for deciding competence is placed on the healthcare practitioner themselves. This is equally true where a role such as prescribing can only be undertaken after successful completion of a recognised course.

If a healthcare practitioner does not consider themselves competent to safely undertake a specific role or task unsupervised, they should not undertake it without that supervision and they need to report this to an appropriate individual, for example the supervisor or line manager. As Cornock (2011) notes, '*it is part of professional accountability to know one's limitations and to be able to accept or refuse tasks and roles based upon whether one feels competent to accomplish them successfully*' (at page 19).

It is important for healthcare practitioners who are expanding their practice, either because they want to do so or because they have been asked to do so, to note that they, the individual healthcare practitioner, are professionally accountable for their practice and any expanded role or task they undertake.

AUTHORITY FROM THE HEALTHCARE PRACTITIONER'S EMPLOYER

Most healthcare practitioners are employed and will have a contract of employment. As well as the usual conditions of employment, the contract of employment will detail the role and duties of the position that the healthcare practitioner has.

Employers are legally entitled to expect that their employees will perform the role and duties as specified in their contracts of employment. What this means for healthcare practitioners wanting to expand their practice is that they need to ensure that they have authority from their employer to undertake the proposed role or task. This authority can be either because it is already in their contract of employment or because their employer has explicitly authorised it as an additional role or task, preferably in writing.

If the employer will not authorise an expansion to the healthcare practitioner's role, and there is no obligation upon them to do so, the healthcare practitioner should not practise outside their specified role. This is because practising outside your contracted role means that you may not be covered by your employer's indemnity arrangement (indemnity arrangements re discussed in **How is an indemnity arrangement related to registration?**).

Healthcare practitioners practising outside of their contracted role and duties may also find themselves in breach of their contract of employment and subject to their employer's disciplinary procedure.

Obviously, this only applies to healthcare practitioners who are employed; if a healthcare practitioner is self-employed, they will be able to make decisions about the scope of their practice themselves, subject to the other requirements in this question.

MEETING REGULATORY OBLIGATIONS

The third requirement is that the healthcare practitioner meets the obligations of their statutory regulatory body.

Essentially this no different to the obligations for any form of practice. The particular requirement for healthcare practitioners expanding the scope of their practice relates to the obligation to have an appropriate indemnity arrangement in place. The key word being 'appropriate'. What may be appropriate for a given role may not be appropriate when that role is expanded in some way.

Healthcare practitioners in employment who have received their employer's authority to expand their practice will be covered by their employer's indemnity arrangement for their normal practice role as well as the expanded role. This is why having an employer's authority is vital before undertaking an expansion of practice.

Q

Why is teamworking a professional issue?

A

As the introduction to this chapter stated, healthcare practitioners do not work in isolation. Most healthcare will be provided through a team approach. Therefore, teamworking, or as it is sometimes known interprofessional working, in healthcare is an essential part of the healthcare practitioner's practice.

There are various definitions of team; the common theme that runs through these definitions is that a team is a number of individuals who have come together to achieve a common objective or outcome or to complete a specified task(s).

The team will be dependent upon each other for the completion of the goal that brought them together. Each member of a team will have an assigned role that contributes to the achievement of the goal. Teams need a team leader; someone who can keep the team working towards the defined goal.

Generally, teams are thought of as being multi-disciplinary, a group of individuals from several different areas of practice, for instance, doctors, nurses, occupational therapists and physiotherapists all working as a team to ensure that patients who are discharged from the hospital setting have the necessary support arrangements in place in their home. Uni-disciplinary teams are also commonplace and are a group of individuals from the same practitioner practice area, such as paramedics. The nurses of a specific ward area are an example of a uni-disciplinary team as they are all working together with the common goal of ensuring that the patients on that ward receive the appropriate nursing care and treatment safely, efficiently and effectively.

Multi-agency teams are those teams where the membership is drawn from different services or from different group of professionals. For instance, a healthcare team is classified a multi-disciplinary team because all its members are drawn for the healthcare professions. If the team were to include social workers and housing officers from the local council, this would have members from outside the health professions and so be a multi-agency team.

The ward team also illustrates another point about teams; it is possible to be part of more than one team at the same time. If we consider student nurse Amelia who works on Fielden ward, Amelia will be part of the nursing team on Fielden ward; she will also be a member of the multi-disciplinary team on Fielden ward, as well as being a member of a specific team looking after a defined group of patents for a shift or couple of shifts before being allocated to a different team caring for a different group of patients on Fielden ward. Amelia may also be a part of a student nurse team at her university working together for a study objective.

Although we can see that Amelia is a member of several different teams, both uni- and multi-disciplinary, her membership of these teams will not all be for the same length of time. Some will be quite transient, such as any shift-based teams, while others will last for a considerable length of time, for instance, any study group team Amelia is a member of for her university course.

Teams are also dynamic in other ways too. Membership can change because a particular individual is no longer available and so another person joins in their place. It is also the case that the shared objective can change as a result of the work that the team has undertaken.

The professional issue in teamwork relates to the fact that, as a member of a healthcare team, you will be working towards a shared objective and the need to ensure that you uphold the professional standard of your profession. Your shared objective is the care and treatment of your patient and, as such, anything you do as part of the team, whether that is a uni- or multi-disciplinary team, a transient, semi-permanent or permanent team, must be undertaken to the same standard as anything else you do in your practice.

This is actually a requirement of the statutory regulatory bodies who have statements in their respective codes of conduct which detail what is expected of a healthcare practitioner when working with colleagues.

Tension can arise in teams, and if this is the case in any of your teams, you will need to ensure that you deal with this in a professional manner. You, and the other members of the team, will be bringing your expertise of your area of practice to the team to achieve the 'goal' of patient care and treatment, and you need to understand your role in the team and work within any constraints that exist, or negotiate a path through the constraints.

It is also important that you understand the roles of the other members of the team and what their unique contribution to the shared objective is, so that you know when to call upon that expertise. Communication is a key aspect of the successful operation of teams. Team members, therefore, need to know the processes that the team is using and what the accepted means of communication is, for instance, are there regular team meetings to discuss progress?

In short, your work as a member of any team should be undertaken to the same professional standard that you are required to achieve in any other aspect of your practice.

Q

If I have concerns about a colleague what should I do?

A

As a professionally accountable healthcare practitioner, you have a duty to raise concerns about a fellow healthcare practitioner's practice or their adherence to their professional standard. Thus, you do not have a choice as to whether to raise any concern you have, as your duty to patient safety and public protection, as outlined in the code of conduct from your statutory regulatory body, overrides any obligation you may feel you have to your colleague. As the Health and Care Professions code of conduct states '*you must make sure that the safety and well-being of service users always comes before any professional or other loyalties*' (Health and Care Professions Council, 2016 at paragraph 7.4).

The key point when raising a concern about a colleague is that you raise it with an appropriate authority. An appropriate authority is one that can take the necessary action. It would not be appropriate to raise a concern about a colleague who is senior to you with someone who is junior to you, as they would be highly unlikely to be able to put any necessary actions in place. It may, however, be reasonable for you to discuss your concerns with a junior colleague to help you finalise your thinking on the issue and what outcomes you wish to achieve.

Most organisations, including NHS employers and universities providing pre-registration courses, will have a policy that details the process to be followed when raising concerns about colleagues, including who the concern should first be raised with. The relevant policy for your organisation should be consulted before you take any action and, where possible, followed. It may not be possible to follow the policy if the colleague you have a concern about is the colleague that the policy states you should be reporting that concern to.

If you are unable to raise your concern according to your organisation's policy, you should discuss this with the relevant department or individual named in the policy, or with your own line manager. The department/individual or your line manager will be able to address your concerns, or they will be able to advise you on the course of action to take, or they themselves will raise your concern with the appropriate authority on your behalf.

There are several routes of support available to you if you do need to raise a concern you have about a colleague. This includes a trade union or professional association if you are a member of one. You can seek the support of your employer's personnel or human resources department. Your colleagues may also be a potential route of support to you. If you are a student healthcare practitioner, you should seek the support of your tutors. As noted above, your line manager, if they are not the object of your concerns, may also be a source of support for you.

See **How should a healthcare practitioner raise their concerns about systems and resources?** for further discussion about raising a concern.

Q How can a healthcare practitioner be a professional and accountable leader?

A A leader is someone '*who guides others in action or opinion*', while leadership is the '*position of leader*' (Stevenson, 2007).

Leadership is an integral part of healthcare delivery both within and outside of the NHS. Without leadership, there would be no development of a strategy to assess and meet future healthcare needs, services and delivery.

Leadership, however, does not just have to occur at the national and strategic level for it to influence healthcare delivery. Local leadership, for instance, at the ward or unit level and at the level of the team (**Why is teamworking a professional issue?** discusses working within teams), is equally vital in ensuing that the healthcare needs of patients are met in a safe and effective way.

The need for a strong level of leadership at local level was recognised in The NHS Plan of 2000 where it was stated that there is a need for '*a strong clinical leader with clear authority at ward level*' (Secretary of State for Health, 2000 at paragraph 9.21). The NHS Plan also reintroduced the matron to the NHS with the introduction of the 'Modern Matron'.

The role of a leader is to lead a team to achieve the objective that they have set or has been set for them. They must be able to inspire a team regarding the objective and the means of achieving it, and motivate individuals as the task continues. Leaders need to use their influence to deal with any disputes that may arise and ensure that challenges do not become obstacles to achieving the objective.

The way that a leader inspires, motivates and influences the team they lead, and the achievement of the objective, will depend upon their leadership style. However, all leaders in healthcare need to ensure that they adopt an approach that meets the standard of their profession. Healthcare leaders are accountable in their own right for the approach they take to their leadership.

Part of a leader's professional accountability will be to ensure that the members of the team they are leading follow their own professional standards. This will in part be met by ensuring that the codes of conduct of the individual team members are adhered to and the team members exhibit professional conduct in achieving the shared objective. The purpose of codes of conduct is discussed in **What is a code of conduct?**, while professional conduct and its relationship to the professional standard is explored in **What constitutes professional conduct?**

While leadership traits are the subject of many books, some of the professional attributes that may be expected from healthcare leader exhibiting a professional standard include:

- Assuming professional accountability for the way the team works and in meeting the objective
- Being transparent and honest in communication within the team and with those outside of the team

- Being realistic about what needs doing and what can be achieved with the resources, including time, available
- Being fair when dealing with members of the team and treating everyone the same, including giving all team members opportunity to participate according to their skills and abilities
- Respecting the members of the team

Q

What is delegation?

A

According to the *Shorter Oxford English Dictionary*, delegation means '*the act of delegating*', and '*a commission given to a delegate*' whist delegate means '*assign or entrust to another*' (Stevenson, 2007).

In healthcare practice, delegation is used when one healthcare practitioner wants another to take on a specific role or task for them. It is very common to delegate aspects of a patient's care and treatment between different members of a healthcare team.

When delegation is employed, it tends to be between healthcare practitioners where there is a position of authority by one of them over the other. This authority may occur because one is higher in the hierarchy, such as a line manager, or because one is a mentor or supervisor to the other or because one is a registered healthcare practitioner and the other is not.

The person with the authority is the delegator and delegates the task to the person without authority who becomes the delegatee. Notwithstanding the authority dynamic between the two healthcare practitioners, the delegatee has to accept the task being delegated for the delegation to have occurred.

An example of delegation in healthcare would be when a staff nurse asks a student nurse to take a patient's blood pressure and pulse hourly for the next four hours while they are receiving a specific intravenous drug and to report back to them if either measurement falls outside a specified set of parameters.

Q

What is referral?

A

Referral according to the *Shorter Oxford English Dictionary* means '*the referring of an individual to an expert or a specialist for advice*' (Stevenson, 2007).

Referral is the basis for many interactions between different healthcare practitioner groups within healthcare practice. It is used when one healthcare practitioner wants the input of another healthcare practitioner in a patient's care and treatment because they lack the specialist knowledge or skills that the latter has. Patients can be referred to another healthcare practitioner for them to take over the entirety of the patient's care or treatment, or for a specific aspect of it with the referring healthcare practitioner still providing the rest of the care or treatment needed.

When referring a patient to another healthcare practitioner, the referring healthcare practitioner does not have to be in a position of authority over the healthcare practitioner they are referring the patient to. Thus, a referral can be made to someone lower in a hierarchy, to someone of equal standing or to someone who is higher in the hierarchy. This is because a referral is a request made to another healthcare practitioner and not an order or demand. The healthcare practitioner to whom the request is addressed must accept the referral for it to have been completed.

An example of a referral is when a nurse asks a physiotherapist to assess the respiratory function of a patient on an intensive care unit and provide any indicated treatment.

Q

What is the difference between delegation and referral for healthcare practitioners?

A

As discussed in **What is delegation?** and **What is referral?**, delegation and referral are two very distinct processes that are used extensively within healthcare practice.

Delegation is employed when a healthcare practitioner, who has the expertise to undertake the task being delegated, wants another healthcare practitioner to take on responsibility for a task. Referral generally occurs when a healthcare practitioner requires the input of another healthcare practitioner because they lack the expertise to do the task themselves.

Referral can occur between healthcare practitioners regardless of any authority relationship between the two. Delegation on the other hand requires the healthcare practitioner doing the delegating to have some authority over the other healthcare practitioner.

Regardless of whether delegation or referral is employed, the healthcare practitioner to whom the request is made needs to accept the delegated task or the referral. The healthcare practitioner to whom the task is delegated or referred has professional accountability for that task.

A major difference between delegation and referral is that with delegation the healthcare practitioner doing the delegating retains professional accountability for the task delegated. This means that two healthcare practitioners have their own, separate, professional accountability for the task. The professional accountability of the healthcare practitioner who delegates the task is to ensure that the task is undertaken and that it is done so in a competent manner, and that they have delegated appropriately. The healthcare practitioner to whom the task has been delegated has the professional accountability to perform the task in appropriate manner and to report any issues and the outcome to the healthcare practitioner who delegated the task to them. When a task is referred by one healthcare practitioner and accepted by another, the professional accountability passes from the referring healthcare practitioner to the healthcare practitioner who accepts the referral.

Both delegation and referral require the healthcare practitioner making the request to do so to a competent healthcare practitioner. Indeed, this is a requirement of the statutory regulatory body codes of conduct. The Health and Care Professions code of conduct states that a healthcare practitioner '*must only delegate work to someone who has the knowledge, skills and experience to carry it out safely and effectively*' (Health and Care Professions Council, 2016 at paragraph 4.1). Similarly, the Nursing and Midwifery Council's code of conduct states that healthcare practitioners must '*only delegate tasks and duties that are within the other person's scope of competence, making sure that they fully understand your instructions*' (Nursing and Midwifery Council, 2018b at paragraph 11.1).

In contrast to referral, delegation requires the delegating healthcare practitioner to supervise the healthcare practitioner performing the delegated task. Again, this is a requirement of the statutory regulatory bodies as outlined in their codes. For instance, the Health and Care Professions code of conduct states '*you must continue to provide appropriate supervision and support to those you delegate work to*' (Health and Care Professions Council, 2016 at paragraph 4.2), with the Nursing and Midwifery Council' code of conduct having a similarly worded provision.

Q

How are registered and unregistered healthcare practitioners different?

A

Using the definitions in **What is a healthcare professional?** and **Is there a legal definition of a healthcare professional?**, a registered healthcare practitioner is a healthcare professional, whereas an unregistered healthcare practitioner is not.

From a professionalism point of view, the difference between registered and unregistered healthcare practitioners relates to their professional accountability. Unregistered practitioners are not subject to the regulatory effects of the healthcare statutory regulatory bodies as outlined in **How does regulation affect the healthcare practitioner?** This includes the fact that as such they do not have to abide by the codes of conduct issued by the statutory regulatory bodies.

Cornock is of the opinion that '*it could be expected that anyone who comes into contact with the patient in a healthcare setting would be subject to the same degree of regulation. However, this is not the case. The regulatory bodies only have jurisdiction over someone who is on the register that they maintain. Anyone who is not on the relevant register is not subject to discipline or sanction by the regulatory body*' (2021, at page 30).

Not being subject to the jurisdiction of the statutory regulatory bodies removes one of the protections that patients have under the regulatory regime overseeing the practice of healthcare practitioners. This explains why unregistered healthcare practitioners must be supervised by registered healthcare practitioners who, by providing that supervision, ameliorate the lack of regulatory oversight of the unregistered healthcare practitioner.

If an unregistered healthcare practitioner is not a healthcare professional, it follows that they cannot have professional accountability for their practice (for an explanation of professional accountability see **Why is professional accountability a key concept in professionalism?**). However, this does not mean that they have no liability for their practice.

Using the categories explored in **Who is a healthcare practitioner professionally accountable to?**, an unregistered healthcare practitioner is liable for their practice to:

- Patients
- Society
- Their colleagues
- Their employers
- Themselves

You will note that they do not have liability to the statutory regulatory bodies, because they are not registered.

The ways in which this liability manifests itself is examined in **Who is a healthcare practitioner professionally accountable to?** and so will not be repeated here.

Q **Is there a difference between mentoring and supervision?**

A Mentoring is generally seen as being a relationship between someone who is experienced and another person who is inexperienced, or at least less experienced. The experienced healthcare practitioner, the mentor, provides guidance and support to the less experienced healthcare practitioner, the mentee.

There is no authority or disciplinary function in a mentorship relationship. Both the mentor and the mentee are equal partners, as the purpose of the relationship is to *'facilitate the personal development and career/professional socialisation for the mentee'* for Morton-Cooper and Palmer (2000 at page 39).

Mentorship relationships can be formal or informal. If it is a requirement for healthcare practitioners working in a specific department to engage with a mentor until they have achieved a prescribed level of competence, this would be an example of formal mentorship.

Informal mentorship occurs when either a healthcare practitioner approached a more experienced collage for their support with working in department x or when a healthcare practitioner notices that a less experienced colleague is in need of support and offers to support them.

There are no guidelines as to how a mentoring relationship has to operate. It is entirely the reserve of the mentor and mentee to establish a relationship that works for them. Equally there is no specific or normal or expected role for the mentor to adopt in supporting the mentee. Morton-Cooper and Palmer (2000) outline several possible roles that the mentor may adopt:

- *'Adviser*
- *Coach*
- *Counsellor*
- *Guide/networker*
- *Role model*

- *Sponsor*
- *Teacher*
- *Resource facilitator*' (page 42)

Supervision needs to be differentiated from clinical supervision. Clinical supervision as examined in **Is clinical supervision related to competence?** refers to a very specific process that is used extensively throughout nursing and midwifery. The problem with supervision and clinical supervision as two different concepts is that supervision occurs in clinical situations and as such is often mistermed clinical supervision.

To return to a quotation made in the earlier question: Butterworth and Faugier note that clinical supervision *'should not be confused with simple managerial oversight ... [and] ... its purpose is to facilitate reflective practice and push toward a patient-centred focus'* (1994 at page 1).

Supervision is concerned with an oversight function. This is when students are supervised during their clinical placements and the supervisor is assessing, either formally or informally, the student's competence, or when a healthcare practitioner has been deemed to need a formal arrangement where their performance can be assessed.

Clinical supervision is more akin to the mentor relationship described above rather than supervision as just described, although clinical supervision for midwives is a combination of the two as there is an oversight function as well as the mentor relationship.

While both mentorship and supervision exist to develop the behaviour, competence and practice of the person being mentored or supervised, the main difference between the two is that supervision has a management element to it and can be used as management tool. This means that hanging over the person being supervised is the realisation that if they 'fail' to achieve what the supervision is in place for, they may face further consequences that may include requiring them to undertake some formal retraining or restricting their area of practice.

Whether a healthcare practitioner is a mentor or supervisor, they need to ensure that they undertake this role as they would any other and bring the professional standard to bear on this aspect of their practice. They should also be mindful of guidance from the statutory regulatory bodies, including the codes of conduct. Where the supervision is of a student, the statutory regulatory bodies have specific guidance to assist supervisors in their role, for instance, *'standards for student supervision and assessment'* issued by the Nursing and Midwifery Council (2018c).

Mentors and supervisors also need to be aware of their responsibilities if the mentee or supervisee gives them cause for concern and what they need to do if this does arise, as explained in **If I have concerns about a colleague what should I do?**

Q **Does following an order as part of a team affect a healthcare practitioner's professional accountability?**

A No, it doesn't. Too short an answer? Let me explain the reasoning behind that.

As the question suggests, many healthcare practitioners believe that if they are working as part of a team, it is the team that is liable for any issues that arise, rather than them through their own professional accountability. This is fallacy as there is no concept of team liability in healthcare practice.

It is also the case that some practitioners believe that, if they were to follow the order or instruction from a manager or person more senior in the hierarchy, the manager is the one who is liable not the practitioner who has received the order or instruction.

Unlike in the past, as explored in **What were the traditional roles of healthcare practitioners?**, there is no expectation that one group of healthcare practitioners will follow the orders of another. Rather each has an equal billing in the provision of care and treatment to patients. As such there is no hierarchy where one can order another to do something they do not want to do. Indeed, all healthcare practitioners must work within their competence and ensure that they meet the professional standard for any task or role they undertake, even when a member of a team.

If a healthcare practitioner does not believe that they are competent to undertake a role or task, they need to state this and ensure that they do not perform that role or task. This was stated as being one of the hallmarks of professional practice in **What is the relationship between professional accountability and competence?** It was stated in **What is clinical competence?** that being competent means knowing when to act and when not to act and that professional accountability is a way of ensuring that healthcare practitioners pay due regard to their competence.

So there is no reason for a healthcare practitioner to follow the orders of another healthcare practitioner unless there is a managerial element to the relationship between the two. Whenever a healthcare practitioner is asked to undertake a role or task as part of a team, they must determine if they are competent to do so. If they are not, their professional accountability requires them to decline the role or task. If they are competent, their professional accountability requires them to undertake that role or task to the expected standard. Whatever they do, it is their professional accountability that will be judged and not that of the team as a whole.

Each member of a team is professionally accountable for their actions, and omissions, when working as part of the team.

Where the task or role is assigned by a manager, the healthcare practitioner still has their own professional accountability for the actions they take. Just because a healthcare practitioner is following a management order or instruction does not remove their professional accountability to practise safely and competently and maintain a professional standard. Equally, the manager will have their own professional accountability. Any order or instruction they give is the same as if they had delegated a task to another healthcare practitioner. As such, they will retain an element of professional accountability for that task, as explained in **What is the difference between delegation and referral for healthcare practitioners?**

SUMMARY

- Traditionally, the relationship between doctors and other healthcare practitioners was one where the doctor issued instructions and the healthcare practitioner followed them. Doctors undertook the role of diagnosing and treating patients and other healthcare practitioners contributed according to their professional speciality, for nurses this was based on caring for patients during their treatment.
- As a result of the policy changes introduced in the 1992 and later and the reduction in junior doctors' hours, the non-medical healthcare practitioner groups saw a blurring of the traditional boundaries that had existed and opportunities for a move away from their traditional roles into roles that had previously been unavailable to them.
- Through their professional representatives, the statutory regulatory body and by responding to opportunities as they presented themselves, healthcare practitioner groups challenged the traditional roles and boundaries that had existed and fundamentally altered the nature of their professional practice.
- Only a few boundaries exist that limit healthcare practitioners' ability to fully expand their practice. These are all legal restrictions that only permit doctors or doctors and midwives to undertake certain roles.
- Healthcare practitioners who wish to expand the scope of their practice need to ensure that they are competent to undertake the expanded role or task; have the necessary authority from their employer to undertake the expanded role or task; and, have the necessary indemnity arrangement in place for their expanded scope of practice.
- Teamworking can be uni-disciplinary, multi-disciplinary or multi-agency. It can be relatively transient or more permanent and requires the healthcare practitioner to work to the same professional standard as any other aspect of their practice.
- Healthcare practitioners have a duty as part of their professional accountability, to raise any concern they have about a colleague to an appropriate authority. This duty is outlined in the code of conduct from the relevant statutory regulatory body.
- A professionally accountable leader is one who meets the standard set by their profession. A professional leader can inspire and motivate a team towards achieving their objective.
- Delegation occurs when one healthcare practitioner requests another to undertake a role or task for them.
- Referral is when one healthcare practitioner asks another for their specialist input into the care or treatment of a patient.
- Delegation occurs between healthcare practitioners when one of them is in a position of authority, whereas referral can occur between any healthcare practitioners.

- Both delegation and referral have to be accepted by the healthcare practitioner to whom the request is made for the delegation or referral to be made. This is because the healthcare practitioner who accepts a delegated or referred task takes professional accountability for it. However, when a task is delegated, the healthcare practitioner who made the delegation also retains professional accountability for the task; this is not the case when a task is referred.

- It is a requirement of the statutory regulatory body codes of conduct that delegated tasks are only made to those who are competent to accept them and also that the delegating healthcare practitioner has to supervise the healthcare practitioner they delegated the task to.

- Unlike registered healthcare practitioners, unregistered healthcare practitioners are not under the jurisdiction of the healthcare statutory regulatory bodies. They must be supervised in their practice by registered healthcare practitioners. Although they do not have professionally accountability, unregistered healthcare practitioners are liable for their own practice.

- Mentoring is a developmental relationship generally between an experienced and less experienced healthcare practitioner. Whereas supervision, which should not be confused with clinical supervision, includes a managerial oversight role for the supervisor.

- There is no concept of team liability in healthcare practice, so individual team members are professionally accountable for their own actions when working as part of a team.

REFERENCES

Abortion Act 1967.

Butterworth, C. and Faugier, J. (1994) *Clinical Supervision in Nursing, Midwifery and Heath Visiting: A Briefing Paper*. University of Manchester: Manchester.

Clarke, A. (1991) 'Nurses as role models and health educators', *Journal of Advanced Nursing*, 16(10): 1178–1184.

Cornock, M. (2008) *Regulation and Control of Health Care Professionals*. Thesis (PhD): Cardiff Law School, University of Cardiff (unpublished).

Cornock, M. (2011) 'Clinical competency in children's nursing: A legal commentary', *Nursing Children and Young People*, 23(10): 18–19.

Cornock, M. (2021) *Key Questions in Healthcare Law and Ethics*. SAGE: London.

Department of Health (1989) *Report of the Advisory Group on Nurse Prescribing* (The Crown Report). Department of Health: London.

Department of Health (1993) *Hospital Doctors: Training for the Future. The Report of the Working Group on Specialist Medical Training* (Chairman: Kenneth Calman – The Calman Report). Department of Health: London.

Department of Health (1999a) *Making a Difference: Strengthening the Nursing, Midwifery and Health Visiting Contribution to Health and Healthcare*. Department of Health: London.

Department of Health (1999b) *Agenda for Change: Modernising the NHS Pay System*. Department of Health: London.

Department of Health (2001) *A Commitment to Quality, A Quest for Excellence – A Statement on Behalf of the Government, the Medical Profession and the NHS*. Department of Health: London.

Department of Health (18 March 2004) *Press Release 2004/0105 'Winterton welcomes first prescribing pharmacists'*.

Department of Health (30 June 2005) *Press Release 2005/0224 'A new era for NHS ambulance services'*.

Department of Health and Social Security (1977) *Extended Role for the Nurse* HC (77) 22. Department of Health and Social Security: London.

Dowling, S., Barrett, S. and West, R. (1995) 'With nurse practitioners, who needs house officers?', *British Medical Journal, 311*: 309–313.

Doyal, L. and Cameron, A. (2000) 'Reshaping the NHS workforce', *British Medical Journal, 320*: 1023–204.

Female Genital Mutilation Act 2003.

Field, D. and Taylor, S. (1997) 'Health and health care in modern Britain' chapter 2, in Taylor, S. and Field, D. (eds) (1997) *Sociology of health and health care*. Blackwell Science: Oxford.

Glover, D. (1998) 'Down with demarcation', *Nursing Times, 93*(31): 37.

Glover, D. (1999) 'Look before you leap', *Nursing Times, 95*(9): 31.

Gold and Others v Essex County Council [1942] 2 All ER 237.

Health and Care Professions Council (2016) *Standards of Conduct, Performance and Ethics*. Health and Care Professions Council: London.

Health and Social Care Act 2001.

Henderson, V. (1966) *The Nature of Nursing*. MacMillan: New York.

International Council of Nurses (1953) *International Code of Nursing Ethics*. Available from the International Council of Nurses website: https://www.icn.ch/

Laird, S. (July, 2004) 'Physiotherapy leads the way', *MedEconomics, 25*: 46–49.

Medicinal Products: Prescription by Nurses Act 1992.

Morton-Cooper, A. and Palmer, A. (2000) *Mentorship, Preceptorship ad Clinical Supervision* (2nd edition). Blackwell Science: Oxford.

Naughton, M. and Nolan, M. (1998) 'Developing nursing's future role: A challenge for the millennium: 1', *British Journal of Nursing, 7*(6): 983–86.

Nursing and Midwifery Council (2018a) *Future Nurse: Standards of Proficiency for Registered Nurses*. Nursing and Midwifery Council: London.

Nursing and Midwifery Council (2018b) *The Code*. Nursing and Midwifery Council: London.

Nursing and Midwifery Council (2018c) *Realising Professionalism: Standards for Education and Training Part 2: Standards for Student Supervision and Assessment*. Nursing and Midwifery Council: London.

Royal College of Nursing (1997) *Continuing Professional Development: An RCN Guide*. Royal College of Nursing: London.

Royal College of Nursing and British Medical Association (1978) *The Duties and Position of the Nurse*. Royal College of Nursing and British Medical Association: London.

Royal College of Nursing of the United Kingdom v Department of Health and Social Security [1981] AC 800.

Secretary of State for Health (2000) *The NHS Plan: A Plan for Investment, a Plan for Reform Cm 4818-I*. The Stationery Office: London.

Stevenson, A. (ed) (2007) *Shorter Oxford English Dictionary* (6th edition). Oxford University Press: Oxford.

Tattooing of Minors Act 1969.

The Nursing and Midwifery Order 2001 (SI 2002/253).

The Social Security (Medical Evidence) and Statutory Sick Pay (Medical Evidence) (Amendment) (No. 2) Regulations 2022.

The Working Time Regulations 1999 (SI 1999/372).

United Kingdom Central Council for Nursing, Midwifery and Health Visiting (1992a) *Code of Professional Conduct* (3rd edition). United Kingdom Central Council for Nursing, Midwifery and Health Visiting: London.

United Kingdom Central Council for Nursing, Midwifery and Health Visiting (1992b) *Scope of Professional Practice*. United Kingdom Central Council for Nursing, Midwifery and Health Visiting: London.

RESPECTING PATIENT RIGHTS

Recognising the rights that patients have in relation to their healthcare needs and giving them their due respect is a key aspect of being a professional healthcare practitioner. This chapter examines these patient rights and considers how healthcare practitioners can assist their patients to achieve their rights.

After identifying what a right is, Chapter 5 considers who has rights in relation to a patient and their healthcare needs, and what these rights may be, before examining some of the rights in greater detail.

The main rights that are examined are those in relation to consent and those related to confidentiality and access to health records. Rights are considered from both the perspective of the adult and child patient.

Because consent is a vital aspect of healthcare, and could be argued to be the fundamental right in relation to respecting patient rights, you will note that a considerable part of this chapter is concerned with answering questions related to rights about consent.

QUESTIONS COVERED IN CHAPTER 5

- What is a right?
- Do individuals have healthcare rights?
- Can a patient demand a specific treatment?
- What rights do family members have?
- Do healthcare practitioners always have to tell the truth to patients?
- Are patient empowerment and advocacy linked?
- How can autonomy and paternalism coexist in healthcare practice?
- What is the right to consent?
- How is consent related to professionalism and accountability?
- What is legally valid consent?

(Continued)

- What is meant by competence?
- How is competence assessed?
- What is meant by information?
- What is meant by voluntariness?
- Are children able to consent?
- Are patients able to refuse treatment that is being proposed for them?
- Is refusal of treatment an option for a child?
- What is the role of those with parental responsibility in relation to a child's healthcare needs?
- Who is a parent and who has parental responsibility?
- In what ways can a patient give consent?
- Does it matter who obtains consent from a patient?
- Is there a difference between consent and assent?
- When is consent legally valid?
- Is it possible for a patient to withdraw consent once treatment has commenced?
- Can a patient self-discharge from a hospital or the care of a healthcare practitioner?
- What is an incompetent patient?
- Do emergency situations change any of the principles of consent?
- When is it possible to treat a patient without their consent?
- What are best interests?
- Why, as a healthcare practitioner, do I need to know about clinical confidentiality?
- What do we mean by clinical confidentiality?
- What information does clinical confidentiality cover?
- When may confidential information be lawfully divulged?
- When should confidential information be divulged?
- What happens if a healthcare practitioner breaches a patient's confidentiality?
- How can a patient access their own health record?
- Are healthcare practitioners allowed to receive gifts from patients?

What is a right?

For the *Shorter Oxford English Dictionary*, a right is defined as an '*entitlement or justifiable claim, on legal or moral grounds, to have or obtain something, or to act in a certain way*' (Stevenson, 2007).

If we unpick this definition, we can conclude that a right is something that can be claimed by someone and that they can claim legal assistance to enforce the right if necessary. The fact that the right can be enforced is very important. If you cannot enforce a right you have then you don't really have a right, but rather an expectation.

A right that is legally enforceable will have the power of the law behind it and as such can be seen as the highest form of right in terms of being enforceable. This is because it is possible to use the power and resources of the courts to ensure that the right is upheld. Where the right has been breached in some way, the person who has the right can make a claim against the person or organisation that who failed to recognise the right or breached it.

One of the more established set of rights that are enshrined in law and cannot be taken away from individuals are those known as human rights. The origins of human rights began in the seventeenth and eighteenth centuries when the state began to provide protection for its citizens in return for certain obligations from those citizens. Often the obligation was to live with certain restrictions, such as adhering to the laws of the society and paying for the protection received in the form of taxation. In addition, the state agreed to uphold specified values or rights that provided additional protection for the citizens. These values, which later achieved the status of formal rights, were those such as not being imprisoned without a trial, the right to own property, and not being subject to slavery.

Over time, these rights became known as natural rights, fundamental rights and/or human rights. After the end of the Second World War, the protection of human rights was seen as being crucial and this impetus resulted in the drafting of the European Convention for the Protection of Human Rights and Fundamental Freedoms in 1950 which was later ratified by the Council of Europe; this later became the European Convention on Human Rights and came into force on 3 September 1953.

The rights contained within the European Convention on Human Rights were incorporated into UK law through the Human Rights Act 1998 which came into force on 2 October 2000. The Act is still in force and continues to provide the following legally enforceable protections:

- right to life
- right not to be tortured
- right not to be subject to slavery or forced labour
- right to liberty and security
- right to a fair trial
- right not to be punished without due legal process
- right to respect for privacy and family life
- right to freedom of thought and conscience
- right to freedom of expression
- right to freedom of assembly and association
- right to marry
- right not to be discriminated against

In summary, a right is an entitlement that can be legally enforced.

Q Do individuals have healthcare rights?

A The fact that some rights are legally enforceable means that there are some rights that are not. So that what someone may think of as a 'right' is in fact an expectation. In healthcare, contrary to popular opinion, there are no universal rights, using the definition of right from **What is a right?** that a right is legally enforceable, available to everyone apart from one. That single right is the right to be registered with a general practitioner.

Registration with a general practitioner is an entitlement that can be enforced. This does not mean that you can register with a general practitioner of your choice, only that if you cannot find one yourself one will be found for you, although this may not be your first choice or the most convenient for you.

The fact that registering with a general practitioner is the only right that can be enforced has led to discussion of rights that do not meet the standard of being legally enforceable but are things that someone <u>should</u> be entitled to and <u>should</u> be able to legally enforce. Some commentators refer to these rights using the terms moral rights or ethical rights. For example, Hawley (2007) states that '*ethical or moral rights are complementary to the human and legal rights afforded by the law. That is, health professionals need to go further than the human and legal rights to ensure that ethical rights are met. Such types of behaviour are sometimes implied in codes and professional standards as required by different professional bodies, and also in various bills or charters of patients' rights*' (at page 59). While Cuthbert and Quallington (2017) are of the opinion that '*moral rights are rights that are associated with the manner in which people are treated ... these rights are much harder to protect as they are not clearly defined and are not always shared by everyone*' (at page 63).

Hawley makes an interesting point when she notes that codes of conduct imply the behaviour that is expected of professional healthcare practitioners in order to ensure that an individual's moral rights are met. As noted in **What is a code of conduct?**, the reason for the existence of codes of conduct is to ensure that registered healthcare practitioners adhere to the accepted standards of behaviour and practice.

With regard to Hawley's statement about moral rights and patient charters, the National Health Service (NHS) across the four countries of the United Kingdom has identified its underlying principles, although each country has identified this separately in different documents, for instance as a charter or set of core principles or a constitution. These set out the rights that a patient can expect when interacting with the NHS.

This last sentence is key to understanding the rights that individuals have in relation to healthcare. Although everyone has the right to be registered with a general practitioner, all the other rights that you may expect someone to have, for instance, treatment on the NHS being provided free at the point of delivery, only exist when that individual becomes a patient.

At the point that an individual moves to being classed as a patient, they achieve additional rights that they did not have beforehand. However, most of these additional rights are qualified rights, that is, they are entitlements but not absolute entitlements. The patient must qualify for the right, and they can be removed under certain circumstances. As an example, the NHS Constitution for England (2021) states that 'you *have the right to receive NHS services free of charge, apart from certain limited exceptions sanctioned by Parliament*' (Department of Health and Social Care, 2021). This is indeed a right you have, but it is a qualified right. It is not something that you can legally enforce (by the way, the part about the limited exceptions refers to prescription charges and payment for eye tests etc.).

The qualification for the right to access services comes two paragraphs later when it is stated that '*you have the right to receive care and treatment that is appropriate to you, meets your needs and reflects your preferences*' (Department of Health and Social Care, 2021). This means that you can access the services provided by the NHS, but only when you have been assessed as needing them, by a healthcare practitioner.

This is why the right to be registered with a general practitioner is a right in the full sense of the definition, one that is legally enforceable. In order to access the full range of NHS services, you need someone to assess that you need those services, that is, the general practitioner who can refer you to the necessary services.

Because of the fact that very few rights in healthcare are absolute, and so always legally enforceable, the professional standard and codes of conduct are vital in maintaining a healthcare practitioner's professionalism and professional account-ability. For it is the healthcare practitioner, through their professional accountability to their codes of conduct, that will uphold the rights of their patients to being treated with respect and dignity while receiving safe and effective care and treatment.

Can a patient demand a specific treatment?

Healthcare practitioners use their expertise and competence to assess a patient's healthcare needs and offer treatment that they consider is appropriate to meet those needs. There are times when the healthcare practitioner may offer the patient more than one proposed form of treatment as each is considered to be appropriate for the patient's needs.

A patient is legally entitled to accept or reject any of the treatments offered to them. In fact, they may reject all of the treatments offered to them. They are also entitled to ask for a second opinion before accepting a treatment that is being proposed. Although the lack of availability of a suitable healthcare practitioner to provide a second opinion may mean that it is not possible to arrange one.

A patient may also ask a healthcare practitioner if they will provide a specific treatment instead of, or in conjunction with, one of the treatment options that the healthcare practitioner is proposing. It is up to the healthcare practitioner's pro-fessional judgement as to whether they consider the treatment option that the patient is requesting is appropriate to meet the patient's needs.

Although a patient may request a specific treatment, many cases that have gone before the courts have established that a patient is only entitled to choose from the treatments being offered to them. They cannot insist upon a particular form of treatment if the healthcare practitioner is not willing to offer it.

Only if the healthcare practitioner considers that there is a benefit to the patient in the treatment being requested should they provide it. Healthcare practitioners are professionally accountable for the treatment that they provide. If they were to provide a treatment that they do not consider to be of benefit to the patient, because the patient requested it, they would need to account for this decision.

Patients are not legally able to demand treatment; therefore, they are not able to demand a specific treatment. The patient's treatment choices are to accept what is being offered to them, choose between treatments if more than one is being offered, or to refuse any or all treatment that is being offered.

Q **What rights do family members have?**

A Before we answer this question, let's firstly dispel a commonly held myth. Here goes: next of kin do not have any legal status. Although patients are often asked who their next of kin is, there is no legal status in law for a next of kin, nor is there any definition of what a next of kin is or who it should be. As Cornock states *'when we ask a patient who their next of kin is, we generally mean who do they want to nominate as the point of contact for healthcare practitioners should the need arise'* (2021, at page 90).

For the purposes of our discussion, the term 'relative' is used in the ordinary sense of the word, as a patient has relatives, as well as the person that the patient would want contacting.

Now to answer the question.

What follows is from the perspective of adult patients, that is, those aged 18 and over. For a discussion of child patients and the rights of their relatives, see **What is the role of those with parental responsibility in relation to a child's healthcare needs?**

There are two specific ways in which a patient's relative has a legal right to be involved with a patient's healthcare needs. Apart from these two occasions, which we will discuss shortly, relatives have no legal rights in relation to the patient's care and treatment. They certainly have no legal power to intervene on the choice of treatment offered to a patient or as to whether a patient should accept or refuse any treatment that is offered.

Any wishes or desires that the relative puts forward as being for the benefit of the patient should be noted, but it is the wishes and desires of the patient that matter. In fact, from a legal perspective, there is no obligation on a healthcare practitioner to involve a relative in any aspect of the patient's healthcare, and this includes providing any information about the patient and their healthcare needs and treatment.

If a relative wants to be involved in a patients' care and treatment, they can do one of two things. They can ask the patient to inform the healthcare practitioners attending them to include them in healthcare discussions, or they can be formally appointed as the patient's legal representative. Other than this, the relative may be treated as only someone that the patient would like to be the point of contact between the healthcare team and their family.

Obviously there are times when the patient may be unable to make decision for themselves, and this is discussed further in **When is it possible to treat a patient**

without their consent? and **What are best interests?.** Where the patient is unable to participate fully in their own healthcare decision-making, relatives may be able to provide the information that is needed to make decisions to meet the patient's healthcare needs in an appropriate way in keeping with the patient's known wishes and beliefs.

So although relatives do not generally have legal rights, there are situations in which it may be desirable to include them in meeting the patient's healthcare needs. Of course, if a patient gives permission for their relatives to receive information and to be included, this allows the healthcare practitioner to discuss the patient's care and treatment with them, although all decisions need to be made by the patient.

The two situations when a patient's relative has a role in the patient's healthcare needs are in relation to mental health care and treatment and in relation to organ donation.

Mental health legislation has requirements for relatives to perform certain functions in relation to patients who are subject to the provisions of that mental health legislation. This does not mean that just any relative can be involved. Those who are involved have very specific functions, such as to be informed of any application to admit the patient, and to make an application for the patient's admission for assessment or treatment or a guardianship application.

The legislation uses the term '*nearest relative*' to indicate who should fulfil the role of relative and the relevant legislation, the Mental Health Act 1983 (section 26) and the Mental Health (Care and Treatment) (Scotland) Act 2003 (section 254), details how to determine who this should be. In the legislation, there is a hierarchy of relatives, and the person who is deemed to be the patient's nearest relative is the living person highest according to the following hierarchy; where two living relatives exist on the same level of the hierarchy, it is generally the older who takes precedence:

(a) *husband or wife* or civil partner (or someone who has been living with the patient for a period of not less than six months as the patient's husband, wife or civil partner unless the patient already has a husband, wife or civil partner);
(b) son or daughter;
(c) father or mother;
(d) brother or sister;
(e) grandparent;
(f) grandchild;
(g) uncle or aunt;
(h) nephew or niece (Mental Health Act 1983 section 26(1)).

In relation to organ donation, the Human Tissue Act 2004 makes provision for relatives to be involved in the decision of whether a person's organs should be used for organ donation. Again, there is a hierarchy of who should be seen as the appropriate relative to act for the person and, according to section 27(4) of the Human Tissue Act 2004, this is the person highest in the following list:

(a) spouse, civil partner or partner;
(b) parent or child;
(c) brother or sister;
(d) grandparent or grandchild;
(e) child of a person falling within (c);
(f) stepfather or stepmother;
(g) half-brother or half-sister;
(h) friend of longstanding.

It is interesting to note that on this legal hierarchy a friend is considered to be a relative for the purpose of the Act, albeit where no living relatives exist to undertake the role.

Q **Do healthcare practitioners always have to tell the truth to patients?**

A This may seem a very odd question to ask. Throughout the answers in the book acting professional and holding oneself professionally accountable have been put forward as vital aspects of working as a professional healthcare practitioner, so why should the question even be asked?

Indeed, if you were to look at the indexes (notwithstanding the issues with indexes explained in the **introduction**) of the current books on the market that deal with ethics for healthcare practitioners, you would find that most do not even include truth telling or its associated ethical principle in the index, nor in the contents. It is obviously so self-evident that the question does not need addressing.

Yet, is it?

The ethical principle of veracity is the principle of telling the truth and is related to Kantianism (Kant and his associated ethical theory is discussed in **What are ethics?**), which proposes that an action like telling the truth is morally obligatory because the action is not associated with an outcome but has an integrity of its own.

It would be expected that a principle as important as this would be included in the codes of conduct from the statutory regulatory bodies. Neither the Nursing and Midwifery Council code of conduct nor the Health and Care Professions Council code contain the word truth. Instead, both discuss the need for the registrant to '*act with honesty and integrity at all times*' (Nursing and Midwifery Council, 2018 at paragraph 20.20) and to '*be honest and trustworthy*' (Health and Care Professions Council, 2016 at paragraph 9).

Being truthful is seen as one of the tenets of building trust, that if someone is untruthful, you are less likely to trust them. Trust is essential to healthcare practice so that patients will engage with the healthcare system and have their healthcare needs assessed and addressed (Cuthbert & Quallington, 2008). Patients need to trust that the healthcare practitioners they engage with are acting in their best interests. Without trust, the relationship between patients and healthcare practitioners may break down.

It is generally accepted that a healthcare practitioner should not lie to a patient; that doing so is unprofessional and will breach the trust that exists between patient and healthcare practitioner. However, there are times when a healthcare practitioner may need to omit some piece of information from their discussion. Is omitting information the same as lying, or is it a separate aspect of veracity?

Tippett (2004) states that while '*debate is ongoing. Some argue that as omission is a failure to act, you are less culpable for an omission than for a lie, as that involves an act of dishonesty*' (at page 3).

It is perhaps opportune to consider why a healthcare practitioner may not want to tell their patients the whole unedited truth. Various reasons and scenarios are stated as reasons not to tell patients the whole truth, and it is generally an omission that is being proposed, certainly no commentator suggests that a healthcare practitioner lies to a patient. These reasons include where:

- a treatment is not available for a patient, there is no reason to raise it;
- a patient asks not to be told a prognosis;
- providing information would distress the patient because they are unable to emotionally or intellectually process the information;
- giving all the information may overwhelm the patient such that they cannot decide upon a treatment choice.

Although these reasons are proffered to justify omitting information in certain circumstances, all commentators agree that healthcare practitioners should inform the patient fully when an error or mistake has occurred with no omissions in the information provided (for more on this aspect see **Why is there a duty of candour? and Is the professional duty of candour different to the duty of candour?**).

It seems to be universally agreed that upholding veracity by telling patients the truth without omission whenever possible is the preferred choice. Yet it is seen that truth telling is not an absolute obligation on healthcare practitioners but is rather conditional.

Campbell et al. (2005) make a very important observation when they state that '*truthfulness is not the bald communication of facts: it is the kind of sensitivity to individual need that knows there is a time to speak and a time to remain silent*' (at page 30). While for Beauchamp and Childress (2013), '*veracity in healthcare refers to accurate, timely, objective and comprehensive transmission of information, as well as the way the professional fosters the patient's or subject's understanding*' (at page 303).

Sometimes upholding the professional standard can mean doing something that seems counter to the standard because it provides a benefit to the patient through either meeting their need for beneficence or non-maleficence (for a reminder about these ethical principles see **What ethical principles are relevant to healthcare practice?**).

What this means for the healthcare practitioner is that the default position is to tell their patient the whole truth where it is possible to do so, but where doing so may cause harm to the patient, it is possible and permissible to withhold information. However, this should be a rare occurrence and needs to be assessed for the individual patient and reassessed as necessary.

One final point: do not lie to your patients; this never meets the professional standard.

Q

Are patient empowerment and advocacy linked?

A

When examining **Why are healthcare practitioners professionally accountable?**, it was noted that one of the reasons that regulation of healthcare practitioners existed was because of a power imbalance between patients and healthcare practitioners. Healthcare practitioners are in a position of power over patients because they have expertise and knowledge that the patient does not have. This means that the patient is at a disadvantage in the healthcare relationship. This is why the professional standard and professional accountability exist in part, to ensure that healthcare practitioners do not use this imbalance to the detriment of the patient.

Patient empowerment is a way of addressing the imbalance between the patient and their healthcare practitioner by ensuring that the patient is at the centre of healthcare interactions. The European Patients Forum (2022) defines patient empowerment '*as a process that helps people gain control over their own lives and increases their capacity to act on issues that they themselves define as important*'.

By empowering patients, they are able to make more decisions about their healthcare needs and to direct the course and outcomes of their healthcare inter-actions. In some ways, patient empowerment can be likened to self-care in that it is the patient who directs their own care and makes decision about what they need and how to meet that need. However, patient empowerment is more than self-care.

Patient empowerment moves self-care on a step or two as the patient is given the tools, including knowledge and skills, to manage their healthcare needs with the support of healthcare practitioners. Additionally, patient empowerment allows patients to know that they are making safe and effective decisions about their healthcare needs and also when they need to access the services of a healthcare practitioner.

True patient empowerment allows the patient to self-manage their healthcare needs but also to know when to seek advice or help, as well as how to access that advice or help, at the time it is needed.

Advocacy is linked to this and feeds into patient empowerment but is different to it.

The *Shorter Oxford English Dictionary* defines advocacy as '*pleading in support of*', with an advocate being '*a person who pleads, intercedes, or speaks for another*' (Stevenson, 2007). Traditionally an advocate is a term for a lawyer who represents their client in court.

Teasdale (1998) succinctly sums up advocacy when he states that '*advocacy is about power. It means influencing those who have power on behalf of these who do not*' (at page 1). Advocacy in healthcare exists because of the power imbalance discussed above. It is not an optional extra for healthcare practitioners as it is a fundamental part of their professional accountability.

The Health and Care Professions Council code of conduct does not specifically mention advocacy but does expect its registrants to *promote and protect the interests of service users and carers* (2016 at page 1). While this is a far ranging obligation on healthcare practitioners, it can be seen to include the requirement for them to speak up on behalf of their patients should the need arise, the very definition of advocacy just presented.

The Nursing and Midwifery Council code of conduct goes further by actually requiring its registrants to act as advocates stating that they must *act as advocates for the vulnerable, challenging poor practice and discriminatory attitudes and behaviours relating to their care* (2018 at paragraph 3.4).

Acting as a patient advocate means giving a voice to the patient who is unable to use their own voice. This may be because they are unconscious, or do not fully understand the issue, or because they are emotionally unable to articulate their needs, or because they are unable to access the correct channel to present their case, or just because the healthcare practitioner is better placed to do it for them.

Being an advocate for a patient could mean speaking up against the accepted norm in an organisation. Gates (1994) provides several negative consequences of healthcare practitioners acting as patient advocates including:

- Emotional closeness with the issue/patient
- Guilt at not being effective
- Guilt at having to report colleagues
- Fear of being scapegoated
- Helplessness

Although Gates also notes that advocacy can be *one of the most positive and rewarding experiences ... [due to] ... the success of the nurse and patient in upholding their rights and/or interests* (1994 at page 74).

Advocacy is about speaking up for others and assisting them in achieving their needs when they cannot. In relation to patient empowerment, it may be that the healthcare practitioner advocates for the patient to be allowed to manage their own care or that the patient's voice is heard during treatment decision-making. Advocating for patients can be a first step in empowering the patient. As time goes by, the healthcare practitioner may need to advocate less as the patient uses their empowerment to manage their own healthcare needs.

How can autonomy and paternalism coexist in healthcare practice?

Autonomy as an ethical principle was introduced in **What ethical principles are relevant to healthcare practice?**. There it was stated that a person is autonomous when they make decisions for themselves that are neither coerced nor subject to the interference of others.

In healthcare when a patient is autonomous, they make the decisions regarding their healthcare needs. This doesn't preclude them from taking advice and listening to the opinion of their healthcare practitioners, but they make the decision based on their own value system and their desires and beliefs about their healthcare needs. The role of the healthcare practitioner is to provide information and advice as requested; it is not to make the decision for the patient or to try and control the decision that is made by influencing the patient towards a certain choice.

Autonomy is related to another ethical principle, that of self-determination. Self-determination is also known as human agency, and it is centred on *'the idea that what it is to be human centres on freedom to exercise reason and to act ... of one's own volition'* (Hugman, 2014 at page 72). Removing or restricting someone's autonomy is, therefore, seen as limiting the essence of what it is to be human. This view of self-determination is shared by both the deontological and utilitarianist ethical theories (deontology and utilitarianism are explored in **What are ethics?**).

It can be seen that autonomy is a key concept within ethics and, within professional healthcare practice, respecting a patient's autonomy is a key value that the healthcare professions proffer. While neither the Health and Care Professions Council's nor the Nursing and Midwifery Council's respective codes of conduct directly mention autonomy or self-determination or human agency, the principles are threaded throughout the codes. There are numerous requirements to respect the wishes and beliefs of patients and assist them in making their own decisions in both of the codes.

When autonomy was first discussed in **What ethical principles are relevant to healthcare practice?**, it was noted that paternalism and autonomy are the opposite of each other. This really does beg the question that is being addressed here, just how the two opposing concepts can coexist.

Paternalism occurs when one person exerts a dominant attitude over another, for instance, when one person knows better than another on a particular matter, usually involving an element of choice. In healthcare, this would be typified by a healthcare practitioner making a decision about an aspect of care or treatment for a patient without involving that patient because they, the healthcare practitioner, know what is best for the patient.

Paternalism was an accepted practice for many years in healthcare. Healthcare practitioners were seen as the experts in healthcare and patients as the passive recipients of their knowledge and expertise and expected to accept the treatments offered to them.

Jackson (2006) neatly sums up paternalism when she states that *'we treat people paternalistically when we take steps to restrict their choices for their own good'* (at page 67). She also encapsulates all that is seen to be wrong with paternalism. If a healthcare practitioner is paternalistic towards a patient, they have removed their autonomy and limited their ability to make their own choice, substituting their own judgement for that of the patient.

Paternalism by healthcare practitioners was not undertaken to undermine patients or their choices. It was done with a belief that, by being paternalistic, the healthcare practitioner was being beneficent to the patient; they were acting for the patient's good. This belief was based on the realisation that healthcare practitioners had access to information, skills and experience that the patient did not. This meant that the healthcare practitioner could make decisions with a view of the whole picture. By being paternalistic, healthcare practitioners could ensure that patients did not make an inappropriate decision.

Indeed, Hugman (2014) argues that the healthcare practitioner's range of knowledge, skills and experience is why the patient seeks their assistance in the first place. However, the danger is that the healthcare practitioner takes over the decision-making to the extent that the patient has no involvement in the decision-making about <u>their</u> condition and <u>their</u> healthcare needs. It is this that prompted the move away from paternalism towards respecting each patient's individual autonomy.

Autonomy in healthcare is centred around giving the patient the information they need to be able to make a real choice. Paternalism would withhold the information on the basis that sharing it with the patient is harmful to the patient, and so the decision needs to be made for them.

Both Hugman (2014) and Jackson (2006) acknowledge that paternalism is not a wrong approach to utilise in healthcare, provided it is used appropriately.

Some patients are unable to make decisions for themselves regarding their healthcare needs, whether this is because of a lack of emotional or intellectual maturity, an abnormality of mind or reasoning, or because they are unconscious. In these situations, decisions must be made for patients. This is the place for paternalism, making decisions for the benefit of the patient. The benefit of paternalism in these situations is that the healthcare practitioner uses their expertise to provide an advantage for their patient without affecting the patient's autonomy.

Paternalism still exists in healthcare today and coexists with autonomy, and indeed needs to do so. It is just no longer the prevailing philosophy for the delivery of healthcare, autonomy being paramount.

What is the right to consent?

In 1999, the Department of Health and Welsh Office defined consent as '*the voluntary and continuing permission of the patient to receive a particular treatment, based on an adequate knowledge of the purpose, nature, likely effects and risks of that treatment including the likelihood of its success and any alternatives to it. Permission given under any unfair or undue pressure is not consent*' (page 67 at paragraph 15.13).

Although this is a very useful and succinct definition of consent, consent has been recognised for a much longer period of time. Consent is a modern embodiment of the ethical principle of autonomy: the right of a person to be self-ruling (see **What ethical principles are relevant to healthcare practice?**).

Specifically, consent is a legal recognition of the right to self-determination that the person is able to make a reasoned decision as to what happens to them and their body. It is a legal recognition because the right to self-determination has been deemed to be such an important principle that there are laws in place that protect the right to make one's own decisions.

Consent is not a single act. A healthcare practitioner should not go and get consent from a patient. As the definition from the Department of Health and Welsh Office states, consent is a '*continuing permission*'. The consent that the patient provides has to endure throughout the treatment process.

The legal recognition of the right to self-determination through the use of consent can be traced to an American case in 1914. In this case (Schloendorff v Society of New York Hospital 1914), it was noted that if a surgeon operated on someone without their consent, they would be committing an assault.

Since then, many legal cases and the Mental Capacity Act 2005 have provided the detail on what criteria must be satisfied for a patient's concert to be considered as legally valid.

For Cornock (2021), '*Consent can be seen to be important for the patient as it provides them with legal recognition for their ethical right of self-determination. For the healthcare practitioner obtaining legally valid consent, that is consent which has been obtained in the correct manner, protects them from both legal action and action by their regulatory body*' (at page 68).

Without the patient's consent, a healthcare practitioner is not able to provide treatment to that patient. Indeed, without their consent, a healthcare practitioner is not able to touch a patient let alone provide treatment. Consent is a vital part of the relationship between healthcare practitioner and patient and a requirement for the provision of treatment.

Q

How is consent related to professionalism and accountability?

A

Consent is a perfect example of a professional issue that embodies the various aspects of professionalism and accountability that have been discussed in the other chapters in this book.

In Chapter 1 **Professionalism**, it was stated that autonomy was one of the four ethical principles that underpin healthcare practice (**What ethical principles are relevant to healthcare practice?**) and that professions have shared values that include these ethical principles.

Consent is based on the ethical principle of autonomy and, in particular, the right to self-determination.

When discussing accountability in Chapter 2, it was noted that one of the reasons to hold healthcare practitioners accountable is because there is a power imbalance between them and their patients (**Why are healthcare practitioners professionally accountable?**), in terms of their knowledge and skills, which the patient needs to determine their treatment.

Consent is a legal mechanism whereby patients can enforce their right to be involved in their treatment choices.

Chapter 3 examined what **Being a professional** entails. One of the main mechanisms that the statutory regulatory bodies can ensure that their registrants are fit to practise is through adherence to the shared values by comparing their practice to the codes of conduct (**What is a code of conduct?**).

The codes of conduct issued by the statutory regulatory bodies all require the healthcare practitioner to ensure that they have a valid consent prior to commencing treatment, for instance, the Nursing and Midwifery Council (2018) require their registrants to '*make sure that you get informed consent and document it before carrying out any action*' (at paragraph 4.2).

While looking at the professional aspects of **Working with others** in Chapter 4, it was noted that each member of a healthcare team is accountable for their own actions (**Does following an order as part of a team affect a healthcare practitioner's professional accountability?**).

Consent is not just a matter of concern for somebody else. It is a patent's legal right, and so the healthcare practitioner who is individually treating the patient or doing so as part of a multidisciplinary team has an equal accountability to ensure that the patient's right and their wishes are respected and upheld.

This chapter, **Respecting patient rights,** is concerned with the rights that patients have and ensuring that these are respected, and hence the patient can rely upon them.

Consent is a patient right. A failure to ensure that a valid consent is in place means that a patient is having their right ignored and their self-determination had been taken away.

Chapter 6 is concerned with **Clinical decisions and patient safety.** Respecting a patient's right to consent is one of the ways in which healthcare practitioners can ensure that the patient's voice is heard in the clinical decision-making process and that it is the patient who makes the ultimate decision regarding their care and treatment.

Finally, Chapter 7 examines what happens **If things go wrong.** If a healthcare practitioner does not ensure that the patient provides a valid consent prior to commencing treatment, they may find that they need to avail themselves of the information in Chapter 7, and could face one of the possible consequences that are outlined there.

Consent is the legal embodiment of a person's right to self-determination. It merges common law, statute law, ethics, professional values, accountability and codes of conduct so that all work together for the benefit of the patient by ensuring that their right is recognised and upheld.

What is legally valid consent?

Legally valid consent is the term used to acknowledge that permission has been obtained from a patient for a specific form of treatment in accordance with the legal requirements currently in place.

You will have no doubt heard the term 'informed consent' used when discussing consent. You may also be wondering why that term is not being used but legally valid consent is being used instead. Legally valid consent, as just defined, is the preferred term because informed consent refers to an ethical principle and an American legal principle, but not one within English law at present.

When discussing ethical and professional principles and issues, using the term informed consent is justified. However, when looking at legal aspects of consent it is not and because there are legal requirements that healthcare practitioners have to meet in obtaining consent from patients, the term used throughout this chapter and book will be legally valid consent.

For consent to be legally valid, three requirements must be met. These requirements have developed through legal cases that have come before the courts to clarify the law on consent and form the basis of the consent requirements in the Mental Capacity Act 2005. The Mental Capacity Act 2005 is the main legislative provision covering consent in the healthcare context.

There are three specific requirements related to:

- Competence
- Information
- Voluntariness

Each of these three terms will be explained in the questions that follow.

What is meant by competence?

Firstly, it needs to be acknowledged that there are two terms, competence and capacity, which, although subtly different, are used interchangeably within the healthcare literature. In this book the term competence will be used.

As noted in **What is legally valid consent?**, competence is one of requirements necessary for consent to be recognised as being legally valid. In relation to consent and healthcare decision making, competence relates to the ability of an individual patient to be able to make a decision, that is, to reach a conclusion as to what is the best outcome for them. However, competence does not only relate to being able to make a decision, competence requires that the patient is able to communicate that decision to the healthcare practitioners treating them.

Deciding whether someone can make a decision on their own behalf is quite complex and from an ethical and legal standpoint raises many issues, such as who should be making the decision, the patient or the healthcare practitioner. Should the patient's decision just be taken at face value, or should the healthcare practitioner assess every patient to determine if they are able to provide their consent or not?

It probably won't surprise you to learn that the ability of patients to be able to make their own treatment decisions has been the subject of many legal cases over the years. However, the Mental Capacity Act 2005 now contains the legal provisions regarding competence and how it is to be applied in the healthcare setting.

Underpinning the Mental Capacity Act 2005 are several principles. The primary principle is that everyone is deemed to be competent to make their own decisions, unless and until they can be shown to lack competence. This means that the legal requirement is not on the patient to prove that they are competent to make decisions but on the healthcare practitioner to prove that the patient lacks competence.

Related to this primary principle is the principle that everyone must be assisted to make a decision and, only if all reasonable steps have been taken to assist the patient, could they be declared to be incompetent, that is, lacking competence to make decisions for themselves. The assistance may be in the form of providing interpreters for those patients who do not have English as a first language, or those who use sign language, so that they understand what they are being told and can use that information to make their decision. It could also be in the form of a communication aid for those patients who are unable to verbalise their decision.

Making a decision that is considered to be unwise or is not one that the healthcare practitioners treating the patient would make does not mean that the patient can be declared incompetent. The patient has the right to make decisions that are best for them regardless of what others think or would do in the same circumstances.

The above discussion is mainly concerned with adult patients. The definition of competence, outlined above, is the same for all patients, but the principle in the Mental Capacity Act 2005 of being competent until provided incompetent is different for adult and child patients, as you will see when considering **Are children able to consent?**.

How is competence assessed?

Following the introduction of the Mental Capacity Act 2005, to assess whether a patient has competence to make decisions, the following two-stage test must be used:

- Is there an impairment of, or disturbance in the functioning of, the patient's mind or brain? If so,
- Is the impairment or disturbance sufficient that the patient lacks the competence to make that particular decision?

Section 2 of the Mental Capacity Act 2005 makes it clear that a declaration of incompetence cannot be made on the basis of the patient's age, appearance, behaviour or condition alone.

The application of the two-stage test is as follows:

Stage 1

First, before deciding whether a patient lacks the competence to make a decision under the Mental Capacity Act 2005, it is necessary to show that the inability to make a decision is caused by '*an impairment of, or a disturbance in the functioning of, the mind or brain*' (section 2(1)), in other words, some form of mental disability.

This is sometimes referred to as the 'diagnostic threshold' aspect of the test. If there is no such impairment or disturbance, the patient cannot lack competence within the meaning of the Mental Capacity Act 2005.

Stage 2

If Stage 1 of the test is met, that is the patient has some form of mental impairment or disturbance, the second stage requires it to be shown that it is the impairment or disturbance that is causing the patient to be unable to make the decision in question. Section 3 of the Act sets out the test for determining whether a patient is unable to decide for him/herself and therefore lacks competence.

This aspect of the test does not focus on the outcome or decision that the patient would make or the consequences of that decision, rather it focuses on how the patient makes their decision; as such it is often referred to as the 'functional' aspect of the test. The fact that a patient makes a decision that others would regard as being irrational or inappropriate does not in itself mean that the patient lacks competence to make that decision. In fact, patients are allowed to make any decision they like with regard to a particular treatment, so long as they are competent to do so.

Section 3(1) of the Mental Capacity Act 2005 provides that a person is unable to make a decision if s/he is unable:

(a) to understand the information relevant to the decision,

(b) to retain that information,

(c) to use or weigh that information as part of the process of making the decision, or

(d) to communicate his/her decision (whether by talking, using sign language or any other means),

You must presume that a patient is competent if they do not have any form of mental impairment or disturbance, or, even if they have some form of mental disability, it does not prevent them understanding, retaining or using the relevant information in making their decision, or to communicate that decision.

When discussing the assessment of competence above, it may have come across as if a patient either has competence or they do not. It is also possible that a patient may have fluctuating levels of competence. If this is the case, treatment decisions should be made when the patient is able to participate in the decision-making process where it is possible to wait for the patient to regain their competence.

A further possibility is that a patient may be deemed to be competent for some treatment decisions but deemed to be incompetent for others. This generally relates to the magnitude of the decision being made. For instance, a patient may be competent to make decisions about their general care arrangements but not whether to have their leg amputated as a complication their diabetes. Their lack of competence may be because they cannot understand the seriousness of not having their leg amputated and the possible consequences that could occur.

A final point regarding assessing a patient's competence is who should be undertaking the assessment? Ideally, the healthcare practitioner who is proposing a specific course of action for the patient should be the one who assesses the patient's competence. However, given the seriousness of the assessment, possibly restricting a patient's right to self-determination, and the actual nature of the assessment itself, any consent should be undertaken with the assistance, if necessary, of someone who is skilled in performing an assessment of competence, for instance, a psychiatrist.

Where a patient has been assessed as being incompetent a detailed record should be made.

What is meant by information?

Having the appropriate information on which to base a decision is a key aspect of any decision-making process. Which is why information is seen as a key requirement in the consent process, as discussed in **What is legally valid consent?**.

The issue related to accountability for the healthcare practitioner who is requiring a patient to make a treatment decision concerns the amount of information that they should provide to the patient.

When discussing **What is legally valid consent?**, it was explicitly stated that informed consent was not a requirement for consent given by a patient to be legally valid. This is because for consent to be truly informed the patient would have **all** the information about their condition, the proposed treatment, any alternatives, and the outcomes and consequences of having the treatment or not having it. Quite simply, healthcare practitioners do not have all this information. They may know that there is a 15% risk of a certain complication occurring for a given procedure, but if a patient asked what that complication would mean for them, they may not be able to fully answer that question. If this were the case the consent would not be fully informed, as the patient would not have all the information.

There are also situations where a healthcare practitioner considers it necessary to withhold information from a patient because disclosing it would be '*seriously detrimental to the patient's health*' (Montgomery v Lanarkshire Health Board [2015] at paragraph 88).

This is why the law does not require 'informed consent'. Rather, there is an expectation that the healthcare practitioner will provide the patient with the information that patient needs in order to be able to reach a decision for themselves. This means that information has to be patient specific. You cannot simply hand out a generic leaflet and expect this to meet your professional obligations in regard to providing information to patients. If a particular patient wants information that the healthcare practitioner would not ordinarily provide, unless there is a risk of harm to the patient in sharing the information, it should be shared with them.

On the flipside, some patients may not want to receive a lot of information and provided it is explicitly made clear that there is information that could be shared and is material to treatment choice, it is acceptable not to share the information. It is about patient choice.

The way in which information is shared with patients is also patient specific, what works with one patient may not work with the next. Information has to be provided to patients in a manner that is appropriate for their needs, for example, in a language they understand, and at level they can comprehend.

The main point to remember, when providing information to patients so that they can make treatment decisions, is that the healthcare practitioner has to meet the patient's individual need and requirement for information.

Q What is meant by voluntariness?

A The final requirement outlined in **What is legally valid consent?** concerned voluntariness. The whole purpose of the consent process is to ensure that patients make their own decisions regarding their healthcare needs, that their self-determination is respected.

Coercion or duress can be applied by healthcare practitioners, but it can also be applied by family members. It occurs when a patient is placed under undue influence to accept a particular treatment, or to refuse a specific treatment or even to refuse all forms of treatment.

If a patient were to consent to treatment, or to refuse treatment due to being coerced or put under pressure, their consent would not be voluntary and so their decision would not be legally valid.

Obviously, it goes without saying that healthcare practitioners should not be putting their patients under undue influence in their decision-making. Where a healthcare practitioner suspects that a patient's consent may not be voluntary, they should discuss this with another healthcare practitioner so that the appropriate steps can be taken to protect the patient.

Q Are children able to consent?

A The word child is not being used in a pejorative sense but as an acknowledgement that the law recognises a patient under the age of 18 as a child (Children Act 1989, section 105).

From **What is legally valid consent?**, we know that there are three requirements for consent to be legally valid. Further in **What is meant by competence?**, it was stated that there is a difference when considering competence in adult and child patients. As the requirements for information and voluntariness is the same for all patients, it is the competence of a child that affects their ability to consent on their own behalf.

Anyone over the age of 18 is automatically competent unless it can be proved that they lack competence (Mental Capacity Act 2005, section 1). The law treats patients under 18 differently and does so based on their age.

Patients aged 16 and over, according to the provisions in the Family Law Reform Act 1969 section 8, are considered as if they were 18 for the purpose of providing their consent to receive a treatment or choosing between treatments.

If a child is under 16, a very different approach to competence is taken. Instead of there being an automatic assumption that the child is competent and the need for this it be refuted if a healthcare practitioner does not consider this to be true, the opposite is the case.

A child under 16 who wishes to exercise self-determination needs to prove that they are competent to do so. The onus has shifted to proving competence where the child is under 16.

In order to prove that they are competent to make a treatment decision, the child has to demonstrate that they have, what has become known as, Gillick competence. The principle is named after the Gillick case (Gillick v West Norfolk and Wisbech Area Health Authority and another [1985]) where it was argued that parents should also provide consent when a child is under 16 but ultimately the case was lost.

You may sometimes see Gillick competence referred to as Fraser competence, but this is incorrect. As a result of the Gillick case, a set of principles known as Fraser guidance was established for treating children under 16 with regard to sexual health matters. Some commentators confuse this guidance and the principles around a child being able to provide their own consent (the Gillick competence principles) and contract the two terms.

If a child can demonstrate that they are Gillick competent, they are legally able to consent for themselves. The child has to demonstrate to the healthcare practitioner that is proposing the treatment that they have the intellectual and the emotional maturity to understand their condition, the proposed treatment and any other treatment options, the consequences of not having the treatment, as well as any possible side effects and complications that may arise, and what the expected outcome is likely to be, that is, that they are Gillick competent. Once they have demonstrated all this, they still need to be able to make a decision and communicate this to the healthcare practitioner.

Proving Gillick competence allows a child to provide a positive consent for a specific treatment at a specific time. If the child is not able to demonstrate that they are Gillick competent, they will not have the right to consent for themselves.

Therefore, albeit through different legal mechanisms, a patient under the age of 18 is able to consent for themselves, either because they have reached the age of 16 or because they are assessed to have Gillick competence. Once the child has provided their consent, this cannot be overridden by anyone else, and it is deemed to be a legally valid consent, thereby allowing the healthcare practitioner to lawfully proceed with the proposed treatment.

Q

Are patients able to refuse treatment that is being proposed for them?

A

If the starting point for the existence of the law around cornet is to recognise protect an individual's right to autonomy and specifically their right of self-determination over their body (see **What is the right to consent?**), it would seem absurd if the patient was only allowed to have the right to consent and not the right to refuse to consent. If this were the case, it would not be a right of self-determination they would be exercising but rather a choice between different forms of treatment.

Thankfully, the patient's right to self-determination is fully protected in the consent laws in the United Kingdom and the patient does indeed have the right to refuse any treatment that is being offered to them, provided that the patient is competent to make a decision (see **What is meant by competence?** for a discussion of competence and how it affects consent).

A healthcare practitioner is only able to provide treatment to a patient when the patient has consented to them doing so. If the patient refuses to consent to a specific form of treatment, or indeed to any treatment at all, the healthcare practitioner cannot provide the treatment that has been refused.

The patient's right to refuse treatment was clearly stated in a legal case in 1992. In that case it was noted that

> an adult patient who ... suffers from no mental incapacity has an absolute right to choose whether to consent to medical treatment, to refuse it or to choose one rather than another of the treatments being offered. ... This right of choice is not limited to decisions which others might regard as sensible. It exists notwithstanding that the reasons for making the choice are rational, irrational, unknown or even non-existent (Re T [1992] at page 652–653).

This judgment from Lord Donaldson means that a competent patient is free to refuse to consent to treatment for any reason they wish and does not have to explain their decision to anyone. The mere act of their refusal is enough to prevent a healthcare practitioner from legally proceeding with that treatment.

The only legal requirement on the healthcare practitioner is that the patient is given the relevant information about why the treatment is being offered to them and the consequences of not having the treatment. Provided the patient has been given this information and is competent to make the decision the patient's decision to refuse treatment has to be respected, regardless of what the healthcare practitioners think and regardless of the possible outcome. Patients are even able to refuse treatments where to do so would result in harm to the patient, including treatment that is considered to be life-saving.

Q
A

Is refusal of treatment an option for a child?

Although it was noted that there is a difference in how the law deals with a child who has attained the age of 16 compared to those who haven't when considering **Are children able to consent?**, when considering the child's right to refuse treatment all patients under the age of 18 have the same legal rights and restrictions.

We know that a child aged sixteen or over and those under 16 who are assessed as being Gillick competent can legally give consent on their own behalf. What is different between the law that governs consent for adults and that for children is that, whereas it is only the adult who can consent on their own behalf, family members having no role or right as explained in **What rights do family members have?**, in relation to children, certain family members do have a role and rights.

Specifically, this role and rights mean that those individuals who have parental responsibility in relation to a child (for a discussion of parental responsibility see **What is the role of those with parental responsibility in relation to a child's healthcare needs?** and **Who is a parent and who has parental responsibility?**) are able to provide consent on behalf of a child.

Someone exercising parental responsibility is legally entitled to consent to treatment for a child at any time, notwithstanding if the child is over 16 and legally entitled to consent for themselves or if the child is under 16 but assessed as being Gillick competent. This means that if the child does in fact refuse to provide their consent, someone exercising parental responsibility could consent instead of the child. This overrides the child's refusal and legally means that the child's refusal is null and void.

So, although the child could technically refuse to consent, their refusal has no legal weight if someone with parental responsibility were to give their consent for the treatment to go ahead.

Consent has been likened to a lock and key, most notably in a legal case from 1991 which considered if a patient aged 15 was able to refuse antipsychotic medication. In that case (Re R 1991), it was stated that if treatment was behind a locked door, to open the door you need a key and this is what consent was, the key to being able to access treatment.

Whereas with adult patients the only key is held by the patient themselves, with child patients there are several keys. These being held by the patient if they are aged 16 or over or if they are assessed as being Gillick competent but also by anyone who has parental responsibility for the child. You only need one key to open the door and, using this analogy, you only need consent from any one person who is legally entitled to provide it. Once you have that consent treatment can legally be provided, even if the other keyholders refuse to provide their key (consent).

Where the child refuses to provide their key (consent) but someone else is willing to provide theirs, the healthcare practitioner has the legal authority to proceed with the treatment, rendering the child's refusal ineffective.

So unlike the consent given by a child aged 16 or over or from a child assessed as being Gillick competent accepting a proposed treatment that cannot be overridden, the refusal of a child of any age can be overridden.

However, just because a healthcare practitioner has the legal authority to proceed with treatment, this does not mean that they are obliged to proceed. Treatment can only be provided where the healthcare practitioner believes it is in the patient's best interests to receive it.

Where there is legally valid consent in place from someone with parental responsibility, but a child is refusing treatment, the healthcare practitioner can go ahead with that treatment against the child's wishes. Alternatively, the healthcare practitioner could try to persuade the child that it is in their best interests to receive the treatment. If the healthcare practitioner is of the opinion that forcing a treatment onto a child who is actively refusing would not be in the child's best interests, they should not proceed with it and explain their reasoning to all parties involved.

Q What is the role of those with parental responsibility in relation to a child's healthcare needs?

A Parents and those with parental responsibility are an exception to the statement in **What rights do family members have?** that relatives have no legal right to be involved in the care and treatment decisions for patients.

Parental responsibility is defined in section 3 (1) of the Children Act 1989 as '*all the rights, duties, powers, responsibilities and authority which by law a parent of a child has in relation to the child and his property*'.

Essentially, the responsibility of the person(s) with parental responsibility is to care for and provide for the child, acting in their best interests, until such time as they are able to do so for themselves, or usually to the age of 18.

There is a myriad of rights associated with having parental responsibility for a child, such as the right to give than a legal name, decide upon their education, raise the child according to a particular religious belief and the right to be with the child. However, with regard to healthcare, the right is to be consulted and to act for the child in the decision-making process.

This includes the right to provide legally valid consent to treatment that is being proposed for the child. This right does not extinguish until the child reaches the age of 18. So as was discussed in **Is refusal of treatment an option for a child?** from the age at which the child becomes able to provide their own consent (either the age of 16 or where they are assessed as being Gillick competent for a specific treatment), the ability to provide a legally valid consent rests with more than one person, unlike with adult patients where it only resides with the competent adult.

Further as seen in **Is refusal of treatment an option for a child?**, a person with parental responsibility has the legal right to override a child's refusal to consent to treatment.

There is often more than one person with parental responsibility for a child, for instance, two parents. Where this is the case the two parents do not have to agree when making treatment decisions for the child. Returning to the lock and key analogy from **Is refusal of treatment an option for a child?**, only one key is necessary to unlock the door, and this could come from anyone with parental responsibility, even if another person with parental responsibility does not agree with the treatment. So theoretically it is possible for the child to refuse to treatment, one parent to refuse but a legally valid consent to be provided by another parent and for the treatment to lawfully proceed.

The only occasions when consent is needed from both parents are when the treatment is not therapeutic, for example, a religious circumcision rather than one needed on medical grounds. Where a decision is being made for a non-therapeutic reason, the consent of both parents is needed and the treatment cannot proceed if one disagrees.

The professional approach to treating a child would be to discuss treatment options with both parents, and with the child where this is appropriate, and to try to gain consensus. However, consent is only legally required from one person with parental responsibility where the child themselves cannot or will not consent, and the treatment is for a therapeutic reason.

If the healthcare practitioner is of the opinion that someone with parental responsibility is not acting in the best interests of the child, any decision made by that individual can be challenged in the courts, as it is the best interests of the child that are paramount, and those exercising parental responsibility must do so in the child's best interests.

Who is a parent and who has parental responsibility?

We can think of a parent as being a natural parent or a legal parent. For the purposes of this discussion, a natural parent is one who has a biological or genetic link to the child, whereas a legal parent is one who has parental responsibility for a child. It is possible to be both a natural and a legal parent; indeed, this is the case for most parents.

A natural parent is one who has provided genetic material for the creation of the child or, from a legal perspective, someone who has borne and given birth to the child even if they do not have any genetic link to the child, as with some surrogacy arrangements.

Given the increase in assisted means of reproduction in recent years, there is some quite complex law on who should be regarded as the parent of a child. For instance, if man donates sperm under the requirements of the Human Fertilisation and Embryology Act 2008, he is not considered to be the father of the child. Subject to certain conditions, if a woman conceives through the use of donated sperm, the resultant child will be considered to be both her and her husband's child. There is a legal presumption that a child born to a married couple is the child of both parents.

For most healthcare practitioners, consideration of the natural parent is rarely an issue and it who has parental responsibility that is of more concern.

As to who has parental responsibility, by law, the natural mother of the child always has parental responsibility, unless this has specifically been removed by an order of a court such as a parental order. Fathers have parental responsibility if they are married to the mother at the time of the child's birth. Female civil partners of the mother will have parental responsibility where the child was conceived by virtue of the provisions of Section 42 of the Human Fertilisation and Embryology Act 2008.

Parental responsibility may also be acquired by fathers who are not married to the child's mother through a 'parental responsibility agreement' with the child's mother and for children born since 15 April 2002 in Northern Ireland, 1 December 2003 in England and Wales and 4 May 2006 in Scotland, if the father's name is entered onto the birth certificate of the child. Step-parents can acquire parental responsibility on entering into a marriage or a civil partnership with someone who has parental responsibility with the agreement of the parent with parental responsibility or by a court order. A second female parent is also able to acquire parental responsibility on registering as a parent, through a formal agreement with the mother of the child or via a court order.

Others who may have parental responsibility include legally appointed guardians, those who are caring for a child under a child's residence order and a local authority when a court order or emergency protection order has been made. If a child is in foster care, it may be necessary to check who actually has parental responsibility as it can be the natural parents, the foster parents or the local authority.

Parental responsibility is not affected by the divorce of the child's parents. It is generally removed from the natural parents on the adoption of a child and transferred to the adoptive parents. If a child is placed in care, the parents usually retain parental responsibility; however, this is likely to be shared with the local authority under whose care the child has been placed. The Children Act 1989 states that it is not possible to surrender or transfer parental responsibility to another, but it is possible to arrange for part of the responsibility to be met by another. This means that it is possible for someone other than those with parental responsibility to make a decision on a child's behalf with the permission of the individual with parental responsibility, for example, a teacher.

Section 5 of the Children Act 1989 states that where someone has care of a child but does not have parental responsibility they may *do what is reasonable in all the circumstances of the case for the purpose of safeguarding or promoting the child's welfare*.

Where someone without parental responsibility is intending to act on behalf of a child, best practice would be for them to discuss this with the person who has parental responsibility, only where this is not possible, such as in an emergency, should they act, or where the matter was a trivial one.

More than one person may have parental responsibility for a child at any one time, as in the case of parents. In such a situation, any of those with parental responsibility may act to meet their responsibility without the agreement of the others, except where this is prohibited by law, as in the non-therapeutic treatment of the child, for instance, religious circumcision of a boy.

Q In what ways can a patient give consent?

A There are two ways in which consent may be said to be obtained, expressly and implied. Although strictly speaking, as we will see, implied consent is not true consent from the patient.

There are two ways in which a patient may expressly provide their consent. This is either in writing or verbally. Even for a major operation, for instance, open heart surgery, consent does not have to be written for it to be legally valid. While your local policy may dictate that consent for all operations has to be written, and it would be inadvisable for any healthcare practitioner to disregard their local policy, there are very few instances where consent has to be written for it to be legally valid. For most circumstances, oral consent is as legally valid as if the consent had been put in writing.

As consent does not have to be put in writing to be legally valid, written consent does not mean that legally valid consent has been obtained. A signed consent form is documentary evidence that there has been a discussion, not that the patient has given legally valid consent. A form that provides evidence that a discussion was had with patient and outlines that discussion, and the patient's decision, is a valid reason for using consent forms.

For consent to be valid, whether written or oral, the consent given must have the necessary qualities of consent about it. These qualities, described as the basic legal principles of consent, have been outlined in **What is legally valid consent?**

One reason for having written, as opposed to oral, consent is that of protection from claims by patients. It can take several years for civil cases to reach court. In these circumstances, it is often difficult to rely upon one's memory, and it is necessary to refer to the patient's medical notes. Having the consent form in the notes does not necessarily mean that legally valid consent was obtained, but it does suggest that there has been some dialogue between the patient and healthcare practitioner and that the patient signed the consent form for some reason. If the consent was obtained orally, it can be difficult to prove that it was in fact obtained at all, especially where it is the word of the healthcare practitioner against that of the patient. It will be a case of who is believed at the time by the court.

Implied consent, as was mentioned above, is not true consent from the patient, but applies in the situation where the healthcare practitioner infers from the patient's actions or demeanour that they do not object to the procedure or treatment (see box below). It is important to note that the patient is merely not objecting to the procedure or treatment; this is vastly different from giving their permission for the procedure or treatment to be performed. Therefore, implied consent should be utilised for minor procedures or treatments only. Silence on the part of the patient should not be taken as implied consent. From a legal perspective, expressly given consent is always preferred to implied consent because it does not rely upon an inference by the healthcare practitioner as to what a patient wants, but an action by the patient to actively state that they wish to have the proposed treatment or procedure.

IMPLIED CONSENT OR NOT?

Mabel (your patient) requires her blood pressure to be taken. As you approach Mabel you inform her that you need to 'take' her blood pressure. On hearing this, she raises her arm, pushes back the sleeve of her nightdress and offers you her arm. You place the cuff around Mabel's arm and proceed to measure her blood pressure. At the end of the procedure, you help Mabel to readjust the sleeve of her nightdress.

At no time do you ask Mabel for her consent and, consequently, at no time does she expressly consent to the procedure. However, what else could you imply from Mabel's actions, other than she did not object to you taking her blood pressure at that time? This is an example of implied consent. It would be appropriate to rely upon it with this type of procedure because there is little or no harm that could befall Mabel, and it is a routine procedure that Mabel has probably permitted on numerous occasions previously.

To turn implied consent into express consent does not involve anything overly elaborate. It would be a simple matter of when approaching Mabel, instead of informing her that you need to 'take' her blood pressure, you rephrase it so that you ask her a question along the lines of, 'Mabel I need to take your blood pressure, is it okay for me to do so?' When Mabel says 'yes that would be alright', you have her expressly given consent.

Q Does it matter who obtains consent from a patient?

A Yes, and no, is the short answer.

Yes, because the healthcare practitioner who is requesting consent from the patient has to be able to determine if the patient's competence needs assessing and to provide all the necessary information that the patient requires in order to be able to make a decision, as well as determining if the patient is voluntarily providing their consent.

It is easy to imagine that patients would expect the healthcare practitioner discussing their treatment options with them, and obtaining their consent, to be the person who will undertake the treatment.

No, because there is no requirement that the healthcare practitioner who obtains the consent from the patient is the one who will actually undertake the treatment. Big caveat here. So long as the healthcare practitioner who obtains the consent from the patient is able to undertake the procedure so that they can fully discuss it with the patient and answer all the patient's questions and requests for information, or, at the very least, they need to be able to provide the patient with all the information which that specific patient requires in order to be able to make a decision regarding the proposed treatment.

However, accountability for ensuring that there is a legally valid consent in place for the treatment rests with the healthcare practitioner who is providing the treatment, who needs to be assured that the patient has provided their consent before commencing the treatment.

Q **Is there a difference between consent and assent?**

A Consent and assent are another pair of terms that are often confused so that they are used as if they are the same thing rather than two disparate and different concepts.

In the healthcare context, consent relates to the permission given by a patient to a healthcare practitioner in order that treatment may be commenced. As noted in **What is legal valid consent?**, consent is a legal process and has specific requirements in order for the consent to be legally valid.

Assent is a more informal process. There are no legal requirements in order for assent to be given by a patient. As such assent does not have any legal status but can be used as an indication of a patient's wishes.

Whereas consent has to be obtained from a competent patient before treatment can be commenced, and the lack of consent from a competent patient means that the proposed treatment cannot be commenced, assent is often used with patients who are not deemed to be competent to consent. It is for this reason that assent is often referred to as a lesser form of consent. However, seeing assent as a lesser form of consent is misleading because there isn't a choice as to whether to use consent or assent. Consent is always to be used where the patient is competent.

Assent is separate from consent though it is used in similar situations, that is, when a healthcare practitioner wants to obtain a patient's agreement to a particular course of action.

Whereas consent is permission, assent is an agreement to something. Some healthcare practitioners see assent as when a patient does not refuse or disagree with a course of action, but this is incorrect. An absence of disagreement is not the same as assent. Neither is merely going along with a course of treatment and not being asked about it. For assent to exist, the patient has to give a positive affirmation, an agreement in some shape or other.

Assent is generally used when a patient is not able to provide their own consent. So the agreement they give does not have legal standing but does indicate that they are supportive of the course of action.

Some of the ways that assent can be used in healthcare practice is with child patients who are under 16 and not deemed to be Gillick competent, or with adult patients who are incompetent for the purposes of consent. In both groups of patients, the use of assent is a way of involving the patient in their care and the decision-making around their care when they are unable to make the actual decisions and provide legally valid consent but have some understanding and are able to agree to a proposed course of action to a greater or lesser degree.

Q **When is consent legally valid?**

A From the preceding questions and answers in this chapter, it can be determined that legally valid consent will have been obtained if:

- it has been given by a competent patient, that is, one over the age of 16 who has not been assessed as being incompetent, or patient under 16 who has been assessed as being Gillick competent;
- who has been given information that is adequate for their specific needs;
- and has been given voluntarily without any undue pressure or duress.

There are some additional points that can be made which also affect if consent is seen as being legally valid. Consent must be obtained for specific treatments or course of treatment. There is no such thing as blanket consent which will cover everything or anything that the healthcare practitioner believes is in the patient's interest to receive. A patient has not consented to any treatment merely by attending a clinic or hospital.

Q **Is it possible for a patient to withdraw consent once treatment has commenced?**

A As well as being able to refuse to consent to treatment that is offered to them, as discussed in **Are patients able to refuse treatment that is being proposed for them?**, patients are also legally entitled to change their minds about treatment that they have agreed to.

The only condition for this is that the patient must be competent at the time that they wish to withdraw their consent. Although the healthcare practitioner would be legally permitted to ask the patient why they want the treatment to stop and to give them information and guidance/advice regarding the benefits of continuing versus stopping the treatment, there is a fine line between providing this additional information and advice and putting the patient under duress to continue with the treatment. The healthcare practitioner needs to ensure they stay on the correct side of the line and do not put the patient under any duress.

If the patient is not competent at the time that they ask for treatment to be withdrawn, they can continue to be treated where the healthcare practitioner is of the belief that it is in the patient's best interests.

The withdrawal of consent, from a legal perspective, is the same as if the consent had not been given in the first place and renders the provision of the treatment to the competent patient unlawful.

When a patient withdraws their consent during the provision of treatment, the healthcare practitioner must use their clinical judgement to assess where it is safe to simply stop the treatment or if the treatment should continue to a point at which it is safe to stop. If the healthcare practitioner is of the opinion that it is unsafe to stop, this needs to be discussed with the patient. Where a treatment needs to continue, as stopping would be unsafe, only the minimum necessary to achieve a safe point to discontinue the treatment should be performed.

Can a patient self-discharge from a hospital or the care of a healthcare practitioner?

In many ways, a patient who wants to self-discharge, sometimes referred to as 'discharge against medical advice', is the same as a patient who wants to withdraw their consent for treatment (as discussed in **Is it possible for a patient to withdraw consent once treatment has commenced?**).

Patients have the legal right to self-determination through the legal process of consent, and this includes discharging themselves from the care of healthcare practitioners who are treating them. Therefore, so long as the patient is competent at the time of self-discharge and there is no legal reason to prevent them, for instance, if they were sectioned under the provisions in the Mental Health Act 1983, there would be no lawful reason to prevent them leaving the care of their healthcare practitioners.

If the patient is not competent at the time that they wish to leave, they can be detained where it is their best interests to do so.

Although the healthcare practitioner should be careful not to restrict the liberty and movement of a competent patient who has indicated their wish to leave their care, they can seek to ensure that the patient is informed about the risks and consequences associated with their leaving care and the benefits of remaining. The healthcare practitioner also has to be cognisant of not putting the patient under duress to stay.

Contrary to what may be indicated on television programmes, there is no obligation on a patient to wait to speak with someone before they discharge themselves, nor do they have to sign any forms to be permitted to leave.

What is an incompetent patient?

An incompetent patient is one who has been assessed as lacking competence according to the criteria and tests laid out in the Mental Capacity Act 2005 (the criteria and tests are discussed in **How is competence assessed?**).

Where the patient is under 16, the situation is slightly different as all patients under 16 are automatically considered to be incompetent unless they are assessed as having Gillick competence.

The legal effect for any patient in being considered incompetent is that, for the aspect of their treatment that they are deemed to be incompetent, they are not able to give a legally valid consent and so can be treated in their best interests or, where they are under 18, with the consent of someone with parental responsibility for them.

Being deemed to be incompetent is a restriction on the patient's right to self-determination.

Q **Do emergency situations change any of the principles of consent?**

A No, if the patient is competent, all of the principles around consent apply even if the patient's need for treatment is an emergency. If the patient is incompetent, the fact that they have an urgent need for treatment does not mean that you can treat them any differently than if they were not in an emergency situation. You still need to follow the principles for the treatment of incompetent patients (see **When is it possible to treat a patient without their consent?**).

If a competent patient refuses treatment in an emergency situation, this is legally the same as if it was a routine non-emergency situation, and their refusal should be respected as discussed in **Are patients able to refuse treatment that is being proposed for them?**.

Q **When is it possible to treat a patient without their consent?**

A If you are dealing with a competent adult, it is not possible to treat them without their consent. Either obtain consent from them or do not provide the treatment.

It is a well-recognised and established principle in English law that no-one can consent on behalf of another person when they have reached the age of 18. Ever. Even if the patient is incompetent. This was confirmed in T v T and another [1988] which considered whether a court could provide consent on behalf of a 19 year old woman who was severely mentally handicapped, it was decided that the court could not provide consent on behalf of this specific patient or for any adult patient.

If the patient is under 18 the principles outlined in **Are children able to consent?** and **Is refusal of treatment an option for a child?** apply. Parental responsibility means that consent can be obtained from someone else, the person with parental responsibility, but only because the patient is under 18.

Although it was just stated that no-one can ever consent on behalf of an adult patient, there is a sort of exception which is not recognised as an exception to this. Let me explain.

If a competent person makes a Lasting Power of Attorney (LPA) and then becomes incompetent, provided the LPA meets the legal requirements (see below), the person acting as the patent's attorney can make treatment decisions for the patient. However, they are not consenting on behalf of the patient but consenting as if they were the patient. A subtle legal difference which means the statement that no-one can consent for someone over the age of 18 remains correct but in effect means that someone can consent for someone else _if_ they are acting for them under the direction of an LPA.

The requirements for an LPA to be valid and legally recognised include that it is signed, witnessed and registered with the Court of Protection, among many others detailed in the Mental Capacity Act 2005. There are two types of LPA, one that covers the patient's financial affairs and another that covers healthcare and welfare. Healthcare practitioners need to make sure that the correct LPA is in place before accepting an attorney's consent for the patient.

For an LPA to be used by an attorney in relation to life sustaining treatment, the LPA must explicitly state that this authority is given to the attorney.

An LPA can only be used after the patient has been assessed as being incompetent. If the patient regains competence, the LPA is no longer able to be used.

Where the patient is over 18, assessed as incompetent and there is no LPA in place, treatment can still be provided to the patient but only under the principle of necessity. The principle of necessity means that the treatment is necessary _'to preserve the life, health or well-being'_ of the patient (per Lord Goff F v West Berkshire Health Authority [1989] at page 565). In the same case, it was noted that the treatment being proposed must be in the patient's best interests. It was stated by Lord Brandon that the _'treatment will be in their best interests if, but only if, it is carried out in order to either save their lives, or to ensure improvement or prevent deterioration in their physical or mental health'_ (F v West Berkshire Health Authority [1989] at page 551). Best interests are discussed further in **What are best interests?**.

To briefly summarise:

- You cannot treat a competent adult without their consent.
- If the patient is a child, consent can be provided against their wishes by someone with parental responsibility.
- If an adult patient is incompetent, consent can be provided on their behalf by someone exercising authority under an LPA which specifically covers the patient's health and welfare.
- If an incompetent adult patient does not have an LPA in place, they can only be treated under the principle of necessity in their best interests.

What are best interests?

A patient's best interests should be readily easy to determine, shouldn't they? And while we are here, is there really a need to discuss best interests, aren't all healthcare practitioners always working in the patient's best interests?

The concept of best interests and what needs to be considered to determine a patient's best interests developed over a number of years through a succession of legal cases where there were incremental enhancements to the principle. One important step was a recognition that a patient's best interests can include anything that has a benefit to the patient and that this includes psychological and social benefits in addition to medical ones, and that anything that contributes to the preservation of the patient's life or health or their well-being in its general sense can be said to be in their best interests (this was in the judgment to the Re MB 1997 case).

Best interests have to be patient specific and should not be used to justify treatment for the convenience of the healthcare practitioners or the patient's family.

The legal requirements governing best interests are now contained with the Mental Capacity Act 2005, where Section 4 has the detailed provisions which must be adhered to.

Best interests involve a consideration of the health situation the patient is in and the available treatment options, but as Jackson (2019) notes, it is more than this and includes '*factors other than the patient's immediate clinical needs, and can also take account of their emotional and welfare interests*' (at page 261). While Herring (2020) states that a consideration of the patient's best interests should include what is known about their present and past beliefs, values, wishes and feelings and any other known factors that the patient would have used in reaching their decision.

In short, determining a patient's best interests in any specific situation involves trying to work out what decision the patient would have made if they were able to and what they would have considered to reach that decision. This is based on all the known information about the patient and their wishes and beliefs and desires and any previous decisions, including refusal of treatment that they have made.

It is sometimes necessary to consult with family and friends of a patient to determine what the patient may consider to be relevant in reaching a decision. However, it should be made clear that the patient's friends and family are not assisting in the decision-making but providing information to those who will be making the decision on behalf of the patent, that is, the healthcare practitioners involved in the patient's care.

If the patient has previously refused to consent to a specific treatment when competent, their best interests are highly unlikely to be met by providing them with that treatment.

Best interests can only be used with patients who are not able to consent for themselves, that is, those who are incompetent. If the patient is able to provide their own consent, a consideration of their best interests is irrelevant as it is their consent, or lack of it, that will determine the treatment the patient receives.

Best interests are also referred to as the best interests standard, the best interests principle or the best interests test. So long as due weight is applied to what the patient would have wanted or it is believed would have wanted, it probably doesn't matter what it is called. The legislation just refers to it as best interests, always in the plural not the singular.

Q **Why, as a healthcare practitioner, do I need to know about clinical confidentiality?**

A Clinical confidentiality is an example of an ethical principle that can be said to be both deontological and utilitarian in outlook.

As a healthcare practitioner, you are expected to practise lawfully and ethically according to any additional requirements stipulated by your statutory regulatory body. Codes of conduct require that you protect the confidentiality of your patients; you need to know what it is you are protecting and why. It is also highly likely that any contract of employment or university and student agreement will have a confidentiality clause regarding patient information gained during the course of your employment or studies built into them. If you were to breach your duty to maintain patient confidentiality, you could in theory be subject to legal, employer, university and/or statutory regulatory body disciplinary action against you.

Additionally, as we will shortly see, there are other compelling reasons why you need to protect patient confidentiality.

We have seen earlier, when discussing the question **What ethical principles are relevant to healthcare practice?**, that patient autonomy is a key ethical principle in healthcare practice. Patient autonomy is concerned with patients making their own decisions relating to their healthcare. Maintaining patient autonomy is a fundamental principle of healthcare practice. Therefore, if a patient wishes the information they provide to a healthcare practitioner to remain confidential, the patient's autonomy should be respected, unless there are compelling reasons for not doing so.

As we know, autonomy is an individual right; it pertains to a particular individual and is for their benefit. However, there is also a public interest or wider principle at stake in maintaining clinical confidentiality. This is based on the rationale of why patients share information with healthcare practitioners and why a healthcare practitioner needs information from a patient.

If we take the last point first, you need certain information from a patient to be able to effectively treat them. Without patient supplied information your job would be much harder, if not impossible. How do you know what condition the patient needs treatment for if you have no information from the patient? Can you provide a certain treatment or medication if you don't know the patient's allergies or current medication?

The patient shares information with their healthcare practitioner for the same reason; they want to receive safe and effective treatment, and they know that providing certain information will assist that. However, patients provide information in the knowledge and expectation that it will only be used for their benefit and will not be shared unnecessarily or with just anyone. This includes relatives of an adult patient, the police, friends of the patient, work colleagues, in fact anyone who is not directly involved with the patient's care and treatment and in need of the information. If they did not believe this, they might be less disposed to provide you with the information that you are asking for. This would have consequences for them in that they may not want to seek treatment at all, or they may seek treatment but be less than forthcoming when asked to provide information. Either situation could result in them not receiving the treatment they need in a timely manner.

There is also a greater impact of individuals not sharing personal information to their healthcare practitioner than just the impact on their own health. This is the impact on public health. If enough individuals do not seek advice or treatment for their illnesses, because they are fearful of what will happen to their personal information, the health of the wider public may suffer as a consequence. The utilitarian argument would be that maintaining clinical confidentiality for individual patients has a positive effect for the wider public.

To provide optimum healthcare to your patients, you need to maintain clinical confidentiality and, in so doing, will be protecting not only the patient in front of you but also the wider public. To maintain clinical confidentiality effectively you need to know what it is, what it covers and when it can be overridden.

Q **What do we mean by clinical confidentiality?**

A If confidentiality refers to information *'not intended for public knowledge'* (Stevenson, 2007), clinical confidentiality must refer to information that is shared in the clinical environment that is not intended to be shared with others, especially the public!

For Allan (2020), *'confidentiality protects information given in confidence. It relates to the non-disclosure of all information that comes to a health practitioner during their relationship with a person who seeks or receives healthcare services'* (at page 51). This view is supported by Cherkassky (2015) who states that *'in practice the duty of confidentiality means that all the information disclosed to a doctor* [any or all healthcare practitioners] *must be kept confidential'* (at page 259).

Clinical confidentiality is also a duty held by healthcare practitioners. As noted in **Why, as a healthcare practitioner, do I need to know about clinical confidentiality?**, this duty arises out of contracts of employment and between students and their educational providers, and in codes of conduct issued by the statutory healthcare regulatory bodies. The duty also arises in law, though specific legislation that covers the disclosing of information such as the Data Protection Act 2018 but also in the Human Rights Act 1998 where the individual's right to privacy exists and in legislation relating to the provision of healthcare such as the Health and Social Care Act 2012. There is also a common law duty of confidentiality.

All in all, quite an extensive set of duties on the healthcare practitioner, all requiring them to keep their patient's information private and protected.

Q **What information does clinical confidentiality cover?**

A Quite a number of legal cases have been considered by the courts in order to reach the current position on what information should be regarded as confidential. In a case involving the model, Naomi Campbell, it was noted that information that concerns a person's private life is confidential information (Campbell v MGN Limited [2004]).

As a result of these legal cases, almost any piece of personal information could be considered to be confidential. The key to determining if a piece of information is confidential or not is in how it was imparted to the healthcare practitioner.

If a patient shares their personal healthcare information in a pub, they cannot expect everyone who hears it to keep it secret. However, if they were to share it as part of a consultation with a healthcare practitioner where they are sharing it so that they can receive appropriate treatment, they can and should expect that it is not widely shared.

An obligation of confidentiality arises when a person shares information with another in circumstances that they, and others, would reasonably consider imposes a duty of confidentiality on the person receiving the information.

For the healthcare practitioner, there is a difference between the basic duty of confidentiality that everyone has and their duty of confidentiality regarding the information they receive as part of their role as a healthcare practitioner. The healthcare practitioner has a higher duty of confidentiality by virtue of their professional accountability.

If the information is already in the public domain, a legal term for 'it is already known by someone else', there is no obligation to keep it confidential as that is already impossible. However, the healthcare practitioner still has a duty regarding who **they** share the information with. This is because the healthcare practitioner's duty is only to divulge information about a patient to those who need to know it and not to share it any wider than that.

To respect the patient's right to confidentiality, the healthcare practitioner should consider all the information they receive from a patient as being confidential and divulge it only when there is a lawful reason to do so.

When may confidential information be lawfully divulged?

Divulging confidential information means sharing it with anyone other than the person who gave you the information and who the information is about. This question considers when a patient's confidential information may be shared; see **When should confidential information be divulged?** for when it should be shared.

There are three ways in which a healthcare practitioner may lawfully divulge confidential information about a patient to a third party (someone other than the patient or the healthcare practitioner).

Whichever means of sharing a patient's information is utilised, only the minimum amount of information required to achieve the purpose for which it is being shared should be shared.

The first lawful way to divulge a patient's confidential information is with the patient's consent. Provided that the patient is competent (see **What is meant by competence?** for a discussion of competence in relation to consent) when they consent to the sharing of their information, the consent acts as a defence for the healthcare practitioner against any possible adverse consequences of sharing the information.

Discussing the need to share their information with the patient, and gaining their consent to do so, is probably the best way to share confidential information. Having the patient's consent to share their information removes the healthcare practitioner's duty to maintain confidentiality. After all, if the person whom the information is about says that you can share it, who can argue with that?

Therefore, whenever possible, obtain the patient's consent before sharing their confidential information.

There is an exception to the laws and principles of confidentiality that exists for healthcare interactions, which is the second lawful way to divulge confidential information. This exception is for information that is shared between members of the healthcare team that are caring for and/or treating the patient. It is an accepted legal practice for members of a healthcare team to share information about patients between themselves and with other healthcare practitioners.

There are two caveats to sharing information with other healthcare practitioners, whether members of the healthcare team or not. These are that the information should only be shared with healthcare practitioners who need the information in order to be able to care for or treat the patient. If a healthcare practitioner has no interaction with the patient, it is hard to justify for sharing the patient's information with them.

The other caveat is that the minimum amount of information that allows the healthcare practitioner to undertake their role for the patient effectively and safely should be shared with them.

The reason that this exception exists is because there is a legal acceptance that when the patient provides confidential information, they are giving implied consent (see **In what ways can a patient give consent?** for an explanation of implied consent) for it to be shared with those who have a clinical need for it.

Confidentiality laws and principles exist to protect the patient's right to keep their personal information private. It is for their benefit that confidentiality is maintained. This leads to the final lawful way to divulge a patient's confidential information; this is when the patient is not competent to make a decision about their information, and it is considered to be in the patient's best interests for the information to be shared.

If the patient is not competent to make decisions regarding their information, they could not be considered able to give implied consent for their information to be shared among the members of the healthcare team looking after them. In these circumstances, it is the patient's best interests as defined in **What are best interests?** that provides the legal and professional authority for the patient's confidential information to be shared among the members of the healthcare team.

A patient's best interests will be revisited in the following question examining when confidential information should be divulged to a third party.

When should confidential information be divulged?

Having just considered when a patient's confidential information may be shared, we now turn our attention to when it should be shared. From a consideration of 'yes, you can if you need to' to 'you have to share this information or you will be failing in your professional duty'.

There are two situations when a healthcare practitioner should share a patient's confidential information. The first is patient related and is centred around their best interests; the second moves away from what is right for the patient to the wider public interest.

As well as ensuring the patient's best interests that all members of their healthcare team have access to the information they need to be able to effectively and safely care for and treat the patient, a patient's best interests may also be served by passing on their information outside of the healthcare team.

Where a healthcare practitioner has a reasonably held belief that one of their patients is being subject to abuse or neglect, they have a professional duty to respond to this. Where the patient is a competent adult and will not consent to their confidential information being divulged, action may be limited to advising the patient regarding the support available to them and how to report their situation to the appropriate authority.

However, where the patient is a child or incompetent, the healthcare practitioner's duty will probably mean informing a relevant person within their organisation as to the situation and discussing the most appropriate course of action. This could include reporting the situation to an outside agency, for instance, the police or social services.

The information that the healthcare practitioner provides to the outside agency should be the absolute minimum that would achieve the aim of ensuring the patient receives the correct support and protection.

Divulging the confidential information of patients in their best interests when they are unable to provide their consent could be said to be in the public's best interests as well as the individual patient's, as it means that society is protecting its vulnerable members.

There are other reasons why a patient's confidential information should be shared in the public interest. These include because it is a legal requirement to do so, for example, the Abortion Act 1967 and Misuse of Drugs Act 1971 both require certain details to be reported to the relevant authorities. Similarly, in limited circumstances, when healthcare practitioners are required to assist the police such as under the Road Traffic Act 1988 and the Terrorism Act 2000.

The police may also obtain a warrant from a court that requires a healthcare practitioner to provide certain confidential information. Assisting the police in the detection of crime can be seen as being in the public interests. However, the warrant will detail what information is to be provided and only that information should be divulged. No more but no less.

As well as divulging a patient's confidential information to protect vulnerable patients and society as whole through adherence to statutory requirements for disclosure and through 'assistance' in police investigations and prevention of crime, the public interest can also be served by protecting individual members of the public.

Legal cases such as W v Egdell and others [1990] have established that healthcare practitioners have a 'duty to warn'. The 'duty to warn' means that where healthcare practitioners are aware that a patient intends serious harm to an individual or individuals, they should divulge confidential information to an appropriate authority who is able to act on the information to protect the individual(s) concerned.

The final circumstance when a healthcare practitioner should divulge a patient's confidential information is when the patient poses a public health risk, for instance, a patient who will not accept treatment or isolate themselves but has a highly infectious disease.

As noted in **Why, as a healthcare practitioner, do I need to know about clinical confidentiality?** protecting a patient's confidential information is in the public interest and should be undertaken unless it is in the public interest for that information to be divulged to an appropriate authority to protect the public.

Q **What happens if a healthcare practitioner breaches a patient's confidentiality?**

A Because confidentiality is a legal, ethical and professional value, any breach of the patient's confidentiality by a healthcare practitioner could result in serious consequences for that healthcare practitioner.

BREACHING A PATIENT'S CONFIDENCE

There are both intentional and unintentional ways to breach a patient's confidentiality. Obviously when a healthcare practitioner intentionally breaches a patient's confidentiality, they know what they are doing and have a reason to do so, even if that reason is not a lawful one. For example, a healthcare practitioner who is passing information about a celebrity patient of theirs to a colleague who is not part of the patient's healthcare team. Or passes the information to a journalist for money. Not that you would do either of these two things.

It is generally the unintentional breaching of a patient's confidentiality that is more problematic, as at the time that the patient's confidentiality is breached, the healthcare practitioner is not aware that they are doing anything wrong, or in fact that they are passing on the patient's information to a third party and thereby breaching their confidentiality.

Some of the ways in which a patient's confidentiality may be breached unintentionally include:

- In the clinical area when using the telephone to discuss the patient with a colleague but in a non-private space, for instance, the nursing station where relatives of other patients are present.
- Discussing patient details outside of the clinical area with a colleague you need to consult with, examples include

  ○ in hospital cafes
  ○ in lifts
  ○ when travelling to and from work on public transport

> - On social media, both in media open to the general public and those only available to specific groups such as student physiotherapists. Photographs of groups of healthcare practitioners in clinical areas can inadvertently contain patient information, on notice boards for example, or even patient faces.
>
> It is important to recognise that you don't have to name a patient to breach their confidentiality; you just have to give enough information so someone can identify who they are. As an example, if the local newspaper had reported a 39-year-old, blue-haired, female weather reporter had crashed their motorbike while holding a parrot, and you mentioned this in the presence of a third party, it would be quite easy to recognise the person you were talking about even without the patient's name.

A healthcare practitioner found to have breached a patient's right to confidentiality may find that they face:

- their employer's disciplinary proceedings for breaking the terms of their contract to keep a patient's information confidential;
- an investigation by their statutory regulatory body for failure to uphold the values in their code of conduct;
- being sued by the patient for the stress and damage they have suffered as a result of the healthcare practitioner passing on their confidential information without lawful reasons to do so.

Passing on a patient's confidential information to a third party without lawful reasons is a very serious abuse of the relationship that exists between patient and healthcare practitioner and, as such, the consequences are serious too.

How can a patient access their own health record?

Patients have several statutes on their side if they want to access their health records, depending upon their reason for wanting to see their health record.

If the patient is making a claim, or considering making a claim, against a healthcare practitioner, hospital or clinic for alleged negligence, the Supreme Court Act 1981 may provide access to their health record. Section 33(2) of this Act provides that, if a patient were to apply to the High Court, it may order someone to disclose what documents they have and to provide these documents to the applicant (the patient) or to the patient's representatives. The High Court has to be convinced that there is a real prospect of litigation commencing before they will order the release of the health record.

If the patient wanted to see a health record that was being prepared on them for employment or insurance purposes, the Access to Medical Reports Act 1988 provides the necessary authority. The right in the Act extends to seeing the report in the health record before it is sent to the prospective employer or insurer, as well as after it has been sent. As well as a right to see the report, the Act also gives the patient the right to stop the report being forwarded to the prospective employer or insurer and to request that the report is amended, if they consider that it is incorrect or misleading in any way, or to have a statement attached to the report if the healthcare practitioner will not alter the report (Section 5).

If the patient has died and their representatives want access to their health record, the Access to Health Records Act 1990 is relevant as Section 3 allows this where a claim may arise as a result of the patient's death. This Act was at one time the main statutory provision relating to access to health records but was superseded by the Data Protection Act 1998, apart from Section 3 as the Data Protection Act 1998 did not provide for access by the representatives of the deceased person's estate. The Access to Health Records Act 1990 covers health records created since 1 November 1991.

The Freedom of Information Act 2000 may be thought to be useful legislation in accessing a heath record held by a public body, that is, the National Health Service. However, health information is not covered in the provisions of the Act as it is personal information.

The above has shown how someone can access health records in specific circumstances. For patients who just want to see their health record for personal reasons, the main statutory provision which allows a patient to access their health record is the Data Protection Act 2018 (DPA), which replaced the Data Protection Act 1998 and allowed the General Data Protection Regulation of the European Union to become law in the United Kingdom.

The DPA provides access to personal data that is being held about someone on request to the controller of that data. From a patient's perspective, personal data includes health records and so this is a means by which a patient can gain access to their health record. The Act requires a controller of data, who has received a subject access request (the term given to someone asking for their own personal data), to provide to that person details of the information that is held about them, along with details of how the information is being processed (used) and a copy of the information. Apart from exceptional circumstances, the controller cannot charge a fee for supplying the information, and it has to be in a format that the subject can understand.

As well as requesting access to their health records, patients also have the right to ask for corrections to be made if there are inaccuracies present.

Although the DPA gives patients wide ranging access to their health records, there are exemptions to this. The most common exemptions are:

- where the healthcare practitioner believes that disclosing the information would cause serious harm to the physical or mental health of the individual or another person;
- where disclosing the information would also disclose information about a third person.

These exemptions apply not only to access under the DPA but to any of the ways, discussed above, that a patient can access their health record. If any aspect of the health record is withheld, this must be explained to the patient.

Before a patient is allowed access to their record, the record needs to be checked to ensure that third party confidentiality will not be breached and that there is no risk of serious harm to the patient or anyone else from the disclosure of the health record to the patient.

A patient may also make a request to a specific healthcare practitioner providing care or treatment to them for access to their health record. It is a judgement for the individual healthcare practitioner as to whether they share their part of the health record with the patient, after considering the two exemptions detailed above. However, they cannot share something that has not originated from them, for instance, entries made by another healthcare practitioner, without that person's express permission. Healthcare practitioners should know their employer's or clinical area's policy on patients accessing their health records.

Although patients are able to access their own health record, a person is not able to access their relative's health record unless the patient gives their consent, or the patient is incompetent and it is in the patient's best interests to share their health record, or parts of it, with their relatives. Someone acting under a Lasting Power of Attorney (LPA) (see **When is it possible to treat a patient without their consent?** for a discussion of LPA) may be entitled to see a patient's health record if it is relevant to their role as the attorney.

A child over 16 may make a request to see their own heath record, as can those under 16 who can demonstrate their understanding of what they are requesting. A person with parental responsibility (see **What is the role of those with parental responsibility in relation to a child's healthcare needs?** for an explanation of parental responsibility) may request to see the child's health record.

Are healthcare practitioners allowed to receive gifts from patients?

Patients are perfectly entitled to exercise their 'right' to reward healthcare practitioners that they recognise as going beyond what was expected, or simply to say thank you for the care and treatment they have received. We need to acknowledge that this is not a right in the same way as the other rights discussed in this chapter. It is more a recognition that this is something patients might choose to do rather than a right that can be enforced through the law.

It is nice when someone wants to recognise the work you do but, although the recognition is generally welcome, healthcare practitioners need to ensure that they follow the correct procedures if a patient wishes to give them a personal gift.

There are several areas of accountability to consider when a patient offers a gift to a healthcare practitioner.

The law would expect that any gift is offered by a competent patient and that, if the patient is incompetent, the gift is not accepted. Also, that the gift is a voluntary offering and not one that has been offered under duress or as a bribe for favourable treatment. Other than that, there is no legal reason why a healthcare practitioner cannot accept a gift from a patient.

The statutory regulatory bodies would expect the same as the law, but some have further expectations. While the Health and Care Professions Council's code of conduct does not specifically mention gifts the Nursing and Midwifery Council code does.

Paragraph 21.1 of the Nursing and Midwifery Council code states registrants must *'refuse all but the most trivial gifts, favours or hospitality as accepting them could be interpreted as an attempt to gain preferential treatment'* (Nursing and Midwifery Council, 2018).

While this is in some ways very clear, only trivial gifts can be accepted, so no Lamborghini then, what amounts to a trivial gift? There is no hard and fast rule here, but many commentators are of the opinion that gifts up to a value of £50 should meet the criteria for being trivial and therefore be unproblematic.

Employers, and universities for student healthcare practitioners, may have policies regarding the acceptance of gifts. Some policies may require that any gifts offered to individual healthcare practitioners are accepted by the employer rather than an individual. Any healthcare practitioner in the favourable position of being offered a gift should ensure that this does not contravene their employer's, or their university's, policy.

There is also the issue of how a gift may be perceived by others. Not only must a healthcare practitioner's practice be professional, but it must be seen to be professional. If the gift could be seen as compromising your professionalism, it should be refused. Examples would be gifts that are given to obtain preferential treatment but may also relate to the nature of the gift itself. A box of chocolates should not be an issue, but gifts of an intimate and personal nature might.

The timing of the gift could be an issue. A gift offered when the patient is leaving care is acceptable, but the gift that is offered while the patient is still receiving care and treatment may be of concern as to the motive behind the gift.

If the gift is given voluntarily, is not intended to gain preferential treatment, is trivial in nature, is allowed to be accepted by an employer or university policy, is not one that could compromise the healthcare practitioner's professional status, the healthcare practitioner may accept the gift.

Whenever a gift is accepted, it would be best practice for the healthcare practitioner to inform their manager of the gift and who it was from; some policies require this to be done. It is best practice because it demonstrates that everything is above board, and the healthcare practitioner is not attempting to hide the gift for some reason.

When in doubt about whether they can accept a gift, the healthcare practitioner should consult their manager or mentor.

If the healthcare practitioner is not able to accept a gift, they should explain this to the patient and politely but firmly decline the gift.

SUMMARY

- A right is something that can be claimed by someone and provides them with the ability to claim legal protection to enforce the right if necessary.
- Most things we think of as rights in healthcare are not legally enforceable and so not a right but an expectation. The only universal right in healthcare in the United Kingdom is the right to be registered with a general practitioner. Other rights begin when the individual becomes a patient. This is one of the reasons why codes of conduct are needed, as they provide the agree standard that patients can expect to receive from healthcare practitioners, even if no legal right exists.
- Patients are not legally entitled to demand a specific form of treatment. A patient's treatment choices are to accept what is being offered to them, choose between treatments if more than one is being offered, or to refuse any or all treatment that is being offered.
- In general, relatives have no legal rights in relation to a patient's healthcare needs and the term next of kin has no legal standing in a healthcare perspective. The two exceptions are in relation to patients who are subject to mental health legislation where a 'nearest relative' has legal rights and obligations, and under organ donation legalisation where a relative may be involved in making decisions about the use of a person's organs for donation.
- Healthcare practitioners should endeavour to always tell their patients the truth without omitting any information. However, there are some occasions where it may be permissible to withhold information from a patient and still meet the professional standard.
- Patient empowerment is about patients having greater control over decisions that affect their healthcare needs. Advocacy is concerned with speaking up for and representing those who are unable to do so themselves. The two are linked but also operate separately, though advocating for a patient can be the first step to patient empowerment.
- Autonomy is concerned with patients making their own healthcare decision with the assistance of the health practitioner who provides information and guidance as appropriate. Paternalism occurs when a healthcare practitioner makes decisions for the patient. Both autonomy and paternalism coexist in modern healthcare practice with autonomy being the paramount philosophy, and paternalism only being used when necessary and when it does not affect the patient's autonomy.
- Within a healthcare context, consent is permission for a specified form of treatment to take place. Consent is a legal mechanism that recognises a patient's ethical right to self-determination and autonomy over their own body.
- Consent is a perfect example of a professional issue that embodies the various aspects of professionalism and accountability that have been discussed throughout this book.

- Legally valid consent refers to consent that has been provided by a patient in accordance with the legal requirements in force at the time the treatment was provided.
- Currently consent is considered to be legally valid when it is provided by a competent patient who has been given information to meet their specific needs and has been given voluntarily without any coercion or duress.
- Competence refers to the ability of a patient to be able make their own treatment decisions and an adult patient is to be treated as competent unless it can be proved, using the criteria and tests in the Mental Capacity Act 2005, that they are incompetent.
- The Mental Capacity Act 2005 utilises a two-stage test to determine a patient's competence. The first stage assesses if the patient has a mental impairment, and the second stage seeks to determine if this mental impairment affects their ability to make a decision, that is, understanding, retaining or using relevant information to be able to make a decision or to communicate their decision to others.
- Information provided to patients has to be patient specific. Patients need to be provided with the information that they require to be able to make a decision.
- Patients should provide their consent voluntarily and without any duress or coercion.
- A child over 16 is able to give consent but a child under 16 has to be assessed as being Gillick competent before they are able to consent for themselves.
- A competent adult patient is legally entitled to refuse any treatment that is offered to them, even if that treatment is thought to be life-saving.
- While a child can technically refuse any treatment that is offered to them, their refusal can be overridden legally by someone with parental responsibility who can consent on their behalf, even in the face of the child's refusal.
- A person with parental responsibility has certain rights and obligations in respect of the child in their care. One of these rights is to act for the child in the healthcare decision-making process.
- There are strict legal criteria as to who is considered to be a parent. Parental responsibility is usually shared between the child's parents, but legal guardians and Local Authorities can also have parental responsibility for a child, either in place of the parents or in conjunction with them. For therapeutic treatments, consent is only required from one person with parental responsibility for it to be legally valid.
- A patient may provide their consent expressly, that is, in writing or verbally, or it can be implied from their actions.
- Consent should ideally be obtained from the patient by the healthcare practitioner who is going to undertake the treatment. If this is not possible, it should be obtained by someone who is able to explain the procedure and answer all the patient's questions.
- Whereas consent is permission for a course of action, assent is agreement with a course of action.
- Patients are able to withdraw their consent legally at any time, and the withdrawal of consent means that any treatment must cease as soon as it is safe to do so.

- Competent patients are able to self-discharge from hospital or from the care of a healthcare practitioner at any time.
- An incompetent patient is one who is not able to consent on their own behalf.
- The fact that a patient requires treatment in an emergency does not change any of the principles of consent and a competent patient's legally valid consent is still required.
- It is possible to treat patients without their consent only in very limited circumstances. These are: child patients where someone with parental responsibility can provide consent, where an incompetent adult patient has a legally valid Lasting Power of Attorney in place, and, in the best interests of an incompetent adult patient under the principle of necessity.
- Considering best interests is a way of trying to determine what the patient may have decided in a specific set of circumstances and what factors the patient would have considered in making their decision.
- Clinical confidentiality is a legal, ethical and professional obligation on the healthcare practitioner. Maintaining clinical confidentiality has important benefits for society.
- Clinical confidentiality is concerned with ensuring a patient's personal information remains confidential.
- Any information that a healthcare practitioner obtains as a result of an interaction with a patient has the potential to be classed as confidential information.
- Confidential information may be lawfully divulged when the patient consents, or between members of the healthcare team treating the patient who need the information to provide that treatment, or when the patient is incompetent and it is in their best interests.
- Confidential information should be divulged when it is in the patient's best interests or when it is in the public interest to do so.
- A healthcare practitioner who breaches a patient's confidentiality without lawful reason potentially faces serious consequences.
- There are statutory provisions which allow a patient to exercise a right to see their own health record.
- Healthcare practitioners need to be mindful of any employer or university policy that may prevent them from accepting a gift from a patient. They also need to ensure that the gift is given voluntarily and not as a way of obtaining preferential treatment, is trivial in nature and would not compromise their professional status before accepting it.

REFERENCES

Abortion Act 1967.
Access to Health Records Act 1990.
Access to Medical Reports Act 1988.
Allan, S. (2020) *Law & Ethics for Health Practitioners*. Elsevier: Sydney.

Beauchamp, T. and Childress, J. (2013) *Principles of Biomedical Ethics* (7th edition). Oxford University Press: Oxford.

Campbell, A., Gillett, G. and Jones, G. (2005) *Medical Ethics* (4th edition). Oxford University Press: Melbourne.

Campbell v MGN Limited [2004] UKHL 22.

Cherkassky, L. (2015) *Text, Cases and Material on Medical Law*. Pearson: Harlow.

Children Act 1989.

Cornock, M. (2021) *Key Questions in Healthcare Law and Ethics*. SAGE: London.

Cuthbert, S. and Quallington, J. (2008) *Values for Care Practice*. Reflect Press: Exeter.

Cuthbert, S. and Quallington, J. (2017) *Values and Ethics for Care Practice*. Lantern Publishing: Banbury.

Data Protection Act 1998.

Data Protection Act 2018.

Department of Health and Social Care (2021) *NHS Constitution for England*. Available at: https://www.gov.uk/government/publications/the-nhs-constitution-for-england/the-nhs-constitution-for-england

Department of Health and Welsh Office (1999) *Mental Health Act 1983 Code of Practice*. The Stationery Office: London.

European Patients Forum (2022) *What Is Patient Empowerment*. Available at: https://www.eu-patient.eu/policy/Policy/patient-empowerment/#:~:text=Patient%20empowerment%20is%20defined%20in,they%20themselves%20define%20as%20important%E2%80%9D

Family Law Reform Act 1969.

Freedom of Information Act 2000.

F v West Berkshire Health Authority [1989] 2 ALL ER 545.

Gates, B. (1994) *Advocacy: A Nurse's Guide*. Scutari Press: London.

Gillick v West Norfolk and Wisbech Area Health Authority and another [1985] 3 ALL ER 402.

Hawley, G. (2007) *Ethics in Clinical Practice*. Pearson Education: Harlow.

Health and Care Professions Council (2016) *Standards of Conduct, Performance and Ethics*. Health and Care Professions Council: London.

Health and Social Care Act 2012.

Herring, J. (2020) *Medical Law and Ethics* (8th edition). Oxford University Press: Oxford.

Hugman, R. (2014) *A – Z of Professional Ethics*. Palgrave Macmillan: Basingstoke.

Human Fertilisation and Embryology Act 2008.

Human Rights Act 1998.

Human Tissue Act 2004.

Jackson, E. (2019) *Medical Law: Text, Cases and Materials* (5th edition). Oxford University Press: Oxford.

Jackson, J. (2006) *Ethics in Medicine*. Polity Press: Cambridge.

Mental Capacity Act 2005.

Mental Health Act 1983.

Mental Health (Care and Treatment) (Scotland) Act 2003.

Misuse of Drugs Act 1971.

Montgomery v Lanarkshire Health Board [2015] UKSC 11.

Nursing and Midwifery Council (2018) *The Code*. Nursing and Midwifery Council: London.

Re MB (An Adult: Medical Treatment) (1997) 38 BMLR 175.

Re R (a minor) (Wardship: Medical Treatment) [1991].

Re T (Adult: Refusal of Medical Treatment) [1992] 4 All ER 649.

Road Traffic Act 1988.

Schloendorff v Society of New York Hospital (1914) 211 NY 125.

Stevenson, A. (ed) (2007) *Shorter Oxford English Dictionary* (6th edition). Oxford University Press: Oxford.
Supreme Court Act 1981.
T v T and another [1988] 1 All ER 613.
Teasdale, K. (1998) *Advocacy in Health Care*. Blackwell Science: Oxford.
Terrorism Act 2000.
Tippett, V. (2004) *Medical Ethics and Law: An Introduction*. Radcliffe Publishing: Oxford.
W v Egdell and others [1990] 1 All ER 835.

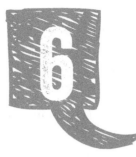

CLINICAL DECISIONS AND PATIENT SAFETY

Decisions are what healthcare is about. Patients want to be able to move forward and need appropriate decision options, but they also want their care and treatment to be safe – this is what Chapter 6 is about.

Decision-making in clinical practice also involves choices made by patients based upon advice and guidance and treatment options provided by healthcare practitioners. It is the decision-making process that leads to these patient choices that is the subject of the first part of this chapter. There is also consideration of the evidence that healthcare practitioners use in the decision-making process.

Chapter 6 examines whether healthcare practitioners are bound to follow guidelines and if they have to record their decision-making, and the value of heath records.

Decision-making is concerned with the right choice being made by patients to meet their own healthcare needs according to their values and beliefs. Healthcare practitioners have their own values and beliefs, and the chapter examines whether they can treat their family and friends, if they can have personal relationships with their patients, and if they are allowed to act according to their conscience when they disagree with certain treatments.

Patient safety is considered throughout the chapter and is specifically considered when looking at the systems within healthcare that exist to improve the quality of healthcare provision, and how safeguarding can act as an additional level of patient safety for those most vulnerable.

QUESTIONS COVERED IN CHAPTER 6

- What is clinical decision-making?
- In what ways can patients have a role in their own healthcare?
- Is shared decision-making the way forward?

- If a healthcare practitioner and patient disagree about the patient's treatment, what should be done?
- What is evidence-based practice?
- How does evidence-based practice relate to being an accountable healthcare professional?
- What constitutes evidence?
- Is there a hierarchy to evidence?
- Do healthcare practitioners have to follow policies and guidance?
- Is it important for healthcare practitioners to record their decisions?
- Can healthcare practitioners treat themselves or their friends and relatives?
- Does conscientious objection absolve healthcare practitioners of their professional accountability?
- What is patient safety and how do risk management, clinical governance and quality assurance contribute to it?
- How does safeguarding relate to patient safety?
- How should a healthcare practitioner respond if they suspect a patient is being abused or neglected?
- Are healthcare practitioners allowed to have relationships with their patients?
- Can patients request a chaperone be present during examinations?

What is clinical decision-making?

Clinical decision-making is undertaken by healthcare practitioners working in clinical practice, and occurs all the time. Because not all the decisions that healthcare practitioners need to make are complex, for instance, the routine (if anything can be described as routine in healthcare) changing of a dressing, many decisions can appear to be made without much thought behind them. As we will see, this is a fallacy and the 'simpleness' of the decision is more about the competence and experience of the healthcare practitioner making that decision than the complexity of the decision being made.

As to what clinical decision-making is and what it encompasses, Standing is of the opinion that '*clinical decision-making is a complex process involving observation, information processing, critical thinking, evaluating evidence, applying relevant knowledge, problem solving skills, reflection and clinical judgement to select the best course of action which optimises a patient's health and minimises any potential harm. The role of the clinical decision-maker in nursing is, therefore, to be professionally accountable for accurately assessing the patients' needs using appropriate sources of information, and planning nursing interventions that address problems and which they are competent to perform'* (2005 at page 34).

As Standing notes, clinical decision-making is a process. A process that is undertaken by healthcare practitioners with the aim of meeting a patient's healthcare needs. Clinical decision-making is not necessarily a once only event. Depending upon the patient's specific healthcare need(s), there may be several clinical decisions to be made at various points throughout the patient's healthcare journey.

The purpose of clinical decision-making is to ensure that healthcare practitioners undertake safe practice, and hence provide safe and effective patient care and treatment.

As well as being a process, as described by Standing above, clinical decision-making is also a balance. This is because the healthcare practitioner has to balance their knowledge, skills, abilities and experience to their understanding of the patient's condition to decide if they have all the necessary information to propose a certain course of treatment. If not, they have to use an appropriate method to obtain any further information they need. This may include deciding to obtain further information from the patient, ordering clinical investigations and/or seeking information about treatment options, including searching for additional evidence and/or seeking assistance from their colleagues.

Once all the information they need is available to them, the healthcare practitioner must balance it to make a decision about the clinical course of action they propose to the patient.

It is this balancing act between a healthcare practitioners pre-existing competence and their acquisition of new information that was being referred to in the opening paragraph of this answer, when it was stated that some clinical decisions can appear to be made without much thought behind them. It isn't that there is a lack of thought behind the clinical decision that is made by the healthcare practitioner, rather that the decision is based more on the healthcare practitioner's pre-existing competence than their need for new information. The healthcare practitioner is able to use their experience of treating and caring for patients with similar issues to make a clinical decision that will meet the needs of the patient before them.

It can be seen that a healthcare practitioner with the necessary experience and competence who is familiar with a certain condition and the treatment for it will be in a better position to propose treatment options to a patient than one who is less experienced and needs to search the available evidence for those treatment options.

Clinical decision-making requires some specific skills from a healthcare practitioner. The healthcare practitioner must be able to learn from experience and apply that experience to current issues. The healthcare practitioner must be able reflect on their previous experiences, including their previous clinical decision-making, so that they can develop their competence by utilising those outcomes that have a positive effect and determine what could have been adapted in those outcomes that did not go as expected. The healthcare practitioner needs to be able to locate and make use of evidence-based information (see **What constitutes evidence?** and **Is there a hierarchy to evidence?** for a discussion of information sources and their reliability). There is a need for the healthcare practitioner to be a critical thinker, someone who can evaluate evidence and information without emotion and with an open mind so as not to prejudge what the final decision will be.

There is also a need for the healthcare practitioner who is making clinical decisions to be an effective communicator. They must be someone who can listen to what the patient is telling them, the way they are speaking about their issues, what they emphasise and see as the important information to impart, as well as being able to determine what the patient is not saying that may be important to their issues. As well as active listening skills, the healthcare practitioner also needs to be an effective provider of information, someone who can impart information to patients and their relatives in a way that is comprehensible to them and means something to them.

Finally, the healthcare practitioner who is making clinical decisions needs to have the ability to share the outcomes from their clinical decision-making with their colleagues, in order to advance the evidence base. As noted in **Why is teamworking a professional issue?**, healthcare practitioners making clinical decisions will be most unlikely to be working in isolation but rather as part of a team. Thus, clinical decision-making requires healthcare practitioners to be effective team members so that patients receive safe and effective care and treatment.

In what ways can patients have a role in their own healthcare?

Patients are at the centre of healthcare practice. The whole of healthcare delivery and the work of healthcare practitioners is focused on patients. Without patients and their healthcare needs, there would be no healthcare delivery and thus no healthcare practitioners. Obviously, there will always be a need for healthcare practitioners as there will always be patients with their attendant needs, but the point is that patients are the core of what healthcare practitioners do.

Various initiatives have been implemented to increase the role of patients in meeting their own healthcare needs. These are often suggested as being new and innovative developments which will enable patients to actively participate in their own care. However, involving patients in their own care is not novel and has been an aspiration for some time with many polices being developed to achieve this over the years, for instance, The NHS Plan of 2000 envisioned '*a health service designed around the patient*' (Secretary of State for Health, 2000 at page 17).

The NHS Plan, when fully implemented, would see patients being empowered to be involved in their healthcare through receiving more information, if they so choose, so that they could make their own treatment decisions with greater choice of how they will be treated. You can be the judge of how far this has been achieved in the 20+ years since it was stated.

Patient involvement in their own healthcare is linked to how empowered they are. The patient who is not empowered or does not feel empowered may not feel that they are able to fully participate in their own healthcare. The healthcare practitioner's role in this situation would include advocating for their patient. The relationship between patient empowerment and advocacy is explored in **Are patient empowerment and advocacy linked?**

When considering the role that patients adopt in their own healthcare, it must be remembered that not all patients are able to be fully involved, for instance, incompetent patients, but also that not all patients want to fully participate.

Thompson undertook a study published in 2007 which examined patient involvement in their healthcare and concluded that here were five levels of involvement. These ranged from absolutely no involvement through to the patient being able to make their own informed decisions.

Information is key to patient involvement in their healthcare. Without adequate information patients will lack the ability to make a fully informed decision. The role of information in decision-making is noted in **What is clinical decision-making?**

There is a possibility that patients may feel overloaded by all the information they need to make a fully informed decision. Some patients may not want to receive all the available information and, as stated in **What is meant by information?**, this is legally and ethically acceptable provided the patient is made aware that there is more information available.

This leads to a crucial aspect of patient involvement in their own healthcare, that patients should only be expected to be as involved as they wish to be. Patients should not be put under pressure to be more involved than they wish and their position not to be as fully involved respected. They should be assisted by the healthcare practitioner as is necessary for the level of involvement they choose.

Where a patient wants to be fully involved in their healthcare, they should be encouraged to do so, receive the appropriate information and, where necessary, have the healthcare practitioner advocate for their participation.

Q

A

Is shared decision-making the way forward?

Shared decision-making is a process. One that aims to reach a decision on how to meet the patient's healthcare needs through collaboration between the healthcare practitioner and the patient. It is a shared process because agreement is reached by both parties contributing to the discussion with the focus on what the patient wants based on the available options.

There are two aspects of shared decision-making which mean that it is an effective way of involving patients in meeting their healthcare needs as well as ensuring patients are supported to reach their self-determination potential:

- Patients and healthcare practitioners are partners in care.
- Patient empowerment and autonomy is to the level that the patient chooses it to be.

PARTNERS IN CARE

Shared decision-making is concerned with ensuring that the treatment the patient receives is best practice focused and tailored to the patient's own values, beliefs, needs and desires.

Patients, in the shared decision-making process, are considered to be the experts with regard to their own bodies, and conditions, and therefore are encouraged and supported to engage in the decision-making by providing their input as they are able.

Rather than the patient being a passive recipient of the healthcare practitioner's guidance and recommendation, the healthcare practitioner needs to ensure that the patient understands all the aspects of their condition, its possible outcomes and consequences, and the various treatment options along with the associated risks and benefits for each, in order to make a decision about what treatment they wish to receive.

Information is key in shared decision-making. If the patient does not have the information or does not understand the information, they will not be able to fully participate in the decision-making process, or will be doing so from a disadvantage. The role of the healthcare practitioner is to assist the patient with the decision-making by providing them with information and support to enable them to make their own decisions. As Wilkinson (2007) states, *'the patient as consumer is entitled to make choices regarding their care and treatment by obtaining the best resources to make an informed choice. It is for the service provider to enter a relationship where they can provide the best insight into the 'product' in this case, care'* (at page 19).

As well as providing the information that the patient needs, the healthcare practitioner should also discuss that information with the patient to assist them in their decision-making. The relationship that Wilkinson writes about is achieved through this providing and discussion of information and choices as part of the shared decision-making process.

EMPOWERMENT AND AUTONOMY AT THE RIGHT LEVEL

Paternalistic healthcare practice, as discussed in **How can autonomy and paternalism coexist in healthcare practice?**, is typified by decision-making that is undertaken by healthcare practitioners, with the patient being a passive participant in the decision-making process. It was also noted that the opposite of paternalistic healthcare is when the patient is fully autonomous and makes all their own healthcare decisions.

There are issues with both of these approaches. In paternalistic practice, the patient has no voice, and decisions are made in their 'best interests', and their self-determination is lost. When the patient is assumed to be autonomous, those patients who do not wish to be fully involved in the decision-making process are nevertheless expected to make their own decisions regardless of their own preference to have less involvement.

When examining **In what ways can patients have a role in their own healthcare?**, it was noted that those patients who want to be fully involved in the decision-making for their healthcare needs should be allowed to, while those who wanted less involved should have this respected. It is shared decision-making that meets the needs of both of these sets of patients. Shared decision-making can be liked to a third approach, or middle way, between paternalistic healthcare and the fully autonomous patient.

Shared decision-making occurs when the patient makes decisions as they want or are able to, and the healthcare practitioner acts as the expert with the knowledge and expertise that they can share with the patient to facilitate the patient's autonomous decision-making. Where the patient wishes to have less involvement, or is not able to fully participate in the decision-making process, the healthcare practitioner can take a more active role in the actual decision-making. For those patients who are unable to have any input into the decision-making, the healthcare practitioner is able to make decisions for them in their best interests.

It is in this way that shared decision-making is a process that is responsive to both patient needs, for instance incompetent patients who are unable to make their own decisions, and to patient wishes, for instance by allowing patients to have as much involvement as they want to have.

Although shared decision-making is the more common term; it is also known as negotiated decision-making and, in some ways, this more accurately describes this form of decision-making as the role of patent and healthcare practitioner is often informally negotiated between themselves as to what part the patient will take in the decision-making process with the healthcare practitioner assuming a lesser or greater role according to the role the patient takes.

Although it has just been said that shared decision-making allows patients to be as active as they want with some taking a more passive role in the decision-making process, the starting point for shared decision-making is that the patient is an active participant. The healthcare practitioner should only assume a greater role when the patient makes it clear that they want to assume a more passive role.

Shared decision-making reduces paternalism in healthcare delivery, increases patient empowerment to the point that individual patients are willing to engage with their own healthcare needs, addresses a patient's lack of knowledge and allows decisions to be tailored to the patient's own beliefs and preferences.

Q **If a healthcare practitioner and patient disagree about the patient's treatment, what should be done?**

A As noted in **What is meant by competence?**, competent patients are entitled to make any decision they want even if the decision they make is one that others do not agree with, or is one that the healthcare practitioner advises against making, or the decision is one that will not lead to an improvement in the patient's condition.

A patient can make any decision they wish for any reason and do not even have to give a reason for their decisions or explain them to anyone else. Making decisions that others do not agree with is not a sign of an inability to make a decision. As the Mental Capacity Act 2005 states, the fact that a patient makes an unwise decision does not mean that they can be assessed as incompetent solely because of that decision.

The issue may be that the patient does not understand the reasons why the healthcare practitioner is suggesting a certain course of action, so the healthcare practitioner may need to provide more information and support to the patient to help them understand this. Any information should be aimed at explaining the reasoning for the choice for treatment and what is hoped to achieve by it and, if there are any, possible alternatives that the patient could have.

If the patient is not aware of the consequences of their decision, the healthcare practitioner should ensure that they discuss the patient's decision with them and clearly highlight the implications of the choice they are making.

Ultimately if, after further discussion, the patient is refusing to have a specific treatment that the healthcare practitioner considers to be in their best interests, then, provided the patient is competent to make the decision, the patient's decision must be respected.

If the patient is refusing treatment that is being offered because they want a specific alternative, the healthcare practitioner should discuss with the patient why they are requesting that treatment, and what they believe it will achieve for them. The healthcare practitioner needs to pay consideration to what the patient says and also if the treatment they are requesting is a viable alternative to the one the healthcare practitioner is proposing. However, if the healthcare practitioner does not consider that the treatment requested by the patient will benefit the patient, they should not provide it. The original treatment option will still be available to the patient, and this should be explained to the patient by the healthcare practitioner along with their reasoning for not offering the patient's choice of treatment. It is then for the patient to consider their options and either accept or refuse those options.

Can a patient demand a specific treatment? stated that patients cannot demand specific treatments that a healthcare practitioner does not think will provide a benefit to the patient.

What is evidence-based practice?

There are almost as many definitions of evidence-based practice as there are forms of evidence. Indeed, there is some debate about what evidence-based practice is and is not. However, most commentators turn to the definition provided by Sackett et al. (1996) which states that '*Evidence based medicine is the conscientious, explicit, and judicious use of current best evidence in making decisions about the care of individual patients. The practice of evidence based medicine means integrating individual clinical expertise with the best available external clinical evidence from systematic research*' (at page 71).

There are two main elements to this definition. The first, which should come as no surprise given it is a definition of 'evidence based practice', is that it requires evidence of some form. The second is that the evidence is no good without the healthcare practitioner's expertise to interpret and use that evidence.

In **Is shared decision-making the way forward?**, it was noted that information is key to the decision-making process. Evidence-based practice is the means of obtaining this information and of making sense of it. There is another aspect of shared decision-making that is relevant to evidence-based practice and that is it is a partnership between healthcare practitioner and patient.

The role that the patient is seen to have in evidence-based practice has been perceived as a criticism of it. If we return to the definition at the beginning of this answer, it should be noted that the patient is nowhere to be seen, apart from as a passive recipient of care and treatment.

The partnership between patient and healthcare practitioner in the patient's care and treatment is seen as so important and one that does need to be recognised as such, that one of the original authors of the definition that is so widely used has supplied a version which acknowledges the patient's role in evidence-based practice. Gray (1997) has stated that *'evidence based practice is an approach to decision making in which the clinician uses the best evidence available, in consultation with the patient, to decide upon the option which suits the patient best'* (at page 3).

Evidence-based practice is a systematic approach to clinical practice which allows the healthcare practitioner to use their expertise and clinical judgement to assess the available evidence to best advise and support the patient in making a decision to meet their healthcare needs.

In many ways, evidence-based practice can be seen as a move away from the paternalistic practices (as defined and discussed in **How can autonomy and paternalism coexist in healthcare practice?**) that used to be prevalent for all patient interactions.

Evidence-based practice is also a quality assurance mechanism. If all healthcare practitioners used an evidence-based approach in their clinical practice, theoretically, provided they are able to effectively assess the evidence, each healthcare practitioner would be utilising clinically effective practice. In short, evidence-based practice should equate to best practice.

By only using treatment that is evidenced as being effective, this should also mean that clinical practice and patient care becomes more cost effective as only those treatments that 'work' are provided.

NOT JUST ABOUT EVIDENCE

It is important to recognise that evidence-based practice, despite its name, is not just about finding evidence to support a particular course of action, nor is it actually just about evidence.

It is about evidence but also about how that evidence is used and the healthcare practitioner's ability to use their expertise to determine what evidence it is appropriate to use to assist their patients in making their decisions.

You may also see evidence-based practice referred to as evidence-based X, where X is the name of a healthcare profession, for example, evidence-based nursing or evidence-based paramedicine.

Q **How does evidence-based practice relate to being an accountable healthcare professional?**

A Healthcare practitioners have a unique set of skills and knowledge that are used to assist patients in meeting their healthcare needs. Because of this, there is a power imbalance between healthcare practitioners and patients, to the disadvantage of the patient, as noted in **Why are healthcare practitioners professionally accountable?**

Holding the healthcare practitioner professionally accountable means that they must be able to justify their actions (see **Why is professional accountability a key concept in professionalism?** for further discussion on this). Another aspect of their practice that healthcare practitioners must be able to account for is their clinical decision-making.

How can a healthcare practitioner justify their clinical decision-making? Gut feeling that treatment X is right? Past experience of using treatment Y? Treatment Z is newer than X and Y so it must be better?

Healthcare practitioners need a rationale for their practice so that they can explain why they made a particular clinical decision. This is where evidence-based practice comes in.

By adopting a systematic approach to clinical decision-making, the healthcare practitioner can point to the evidence they used when making a particular decision if ever called to account.

The healthcare practitioner who adopts evidence-based practice can demonstrate how they have used their clinical expertise and judgement by using appropriate evidence to make best use of the available resources to meet the patient's healthcare needs while also respecting the patient's personal values.

Professional healthcare practitioners recognise that clinical decisions they make have an effect beyond the patient they are assisting. Evidence-based practice allows best practice to be communicated widely, based on sharing evidence of what has had favourable outcomes in specific circumstances and for particular patients. This means that other healthcare practitioners working in the same clinical speciality can adopt those processes when appropriate to do so, thus fulfilling the healthcare practitioner's duty to the wider profession and the sharing of knowledge.

In addition, it is a requirement of the statutory regulatory bodies that healthcare practitioners '*always practise in line with the best available evidence*' (Nursing and Midwifery Council, 2018, at paragraph 6).

Q **What constitutes evidence?**

A The National Institute for Health and Care Excellence (2022) defines evidence as '*information on which a decision or recommendation is based*' (in the glossary). This is not as facile as it may at first seem. It is actually a very useful definition as it recognises that almost anything could be used as evidence for clinical decision-making.

Lamont (2021) acknowledges the difficulty in determining what constitutes evidence when she states that *'it is not always obvious what is seen as valid evidence. Different stakeholders have different needs and value different kinds of information'* (at page 25).

Types of evidence available to healthcare practitioners to use in their clinical decision-making with patients include:

- Anecdotal accounts
- Articles
- Books
- Case reports
- Clinical guidelines
- Conference papers and proceedings
- Department of Health papers
- Employer policies and procedures
- Hospital guidelines
- Internet searches
- Interviews
- Literature reviews
- Media reports
- Meta analyses
- National Inquiry reports
- National Policies
- Patient experiences
- Randomised controlled trials
- Royal College guidance and protocols
- Statutory regulatory body guidance
- Surveys
- Systematic reviews

If almost anything could be used as evidence, and evidence changes according to the reason it is being used, then the healthcare practitioner's expertise and judgement is crucial in determining where to obtain evidence, what evidence is useful and what value to put on that evidence. This is because it is unlikely that patients will have the skill to do this for themselves.

Birrell Ivory (2021) can be seen to support this view of the importance of the role of the healthcare practitioner in finding, selecting and determining which evidence to use, when she states that *'being able to identify different types of evidence, make judgements about their reliability and credibility, and decide when evidence is needed to support our arguments is essential'* (at page 97).

Knowing what evidence to use in a particular clinical situation means that the healthcare practitioner needs to be aware of the evidence available. This necessitates a degree of keeping themselves up to date, for a discussion of how current a healthcare practitioner needs to be see **How up to date do I need to be?** Continuing professional development (for a discussion of what this may entail see **What is continuing professional development?**) is a mechanism by which healthcare practitioners can update themselves about developments in their area of clinical practice.

Is there a hierarchy to evidence?

This is one of those yes and no answers.

Yes, there are differences in the evidence that will be available. And yes, this difference will result in a hierarchy to evidence, based on the reliability that the evidence has. Usually, the more reliability that a piece of evidence has the more weight that can be given to it in providing support for a particular clinical decision. For instance, generally an international clinical trial is more reliable than a national trial which is more reliable than a local trial as the numbers will be larger in the first compared to the second and the second compared to the third.

Primary research is preferred to secondary research, and research as a whole is more reliable than anecdotal evidence. Indeed, the list of evidence presented in **What constitutes evidence?** could be ranked according to which is more reliable than the others. However, reliability is related to usefulness. Therefore, as Lamont (2021) noted, any hierarchy is going to be dependent upon the purpose that the evidence is going to be used for. Taking the example above about clinical trials, if an international clinical trial and a local trial were both available, generally the international trial should be given more weight. However, it may be that the local trial has the greater relevance because of some local factor that is not included in the international trial.

Hierarchies of evidence are useful to see the value of one form of evidence over another, but they have their limitations, and it is the use of the evidence which should determine its value compared to another piece of evidence, not just where it sits in a list.

Do healthcare practitioners have to follow policies and guidance?

We could start this answer by looking at what a policy is and what guidelines are, but that would not be particularly useful because although a policy is something that a healthcare practitioner is expected to follow and a guideline is generally seen as guidance, a national guideline which contradicts a local policy may have more weight to it. Instead, policies and guidance are going to be used as shorthand for all the information that is directed at healthcare practitioners that they are expected to pay attention to and to 'follow'.

Using this shorthand, one way to answer the question is to consider what the potential consequences are for not following policies and guidance. An example to illustrate this would be the policies and guidance around consent. As we saw in Chapter 5, **Respecting patient rights**, consent is a vital part of the healthcare process and because of this there is a lot of information available.

There are four categories into which policies and guidance can be categorised:

- Legal
- Regulatory
- Professional
- Other, including employer issued and more general information

Reviewing the answers addressing consent in Chapter 5, **Respecting patient rights**, the following are examples of the information that can be identified under each of the four categories above.

LEGAL

Statutes such as the Children Act 1989 and the Mental Capacity Act 2005.
Legal cases including Montgomery v Lanarkshire Health Board [2015] and Gillick v West Norfolk and Wisbech Area Health Authority and another [1985].

REGULATORY

The Health and Care Professions Council (2016) *Standards of conduct, performance and ethics* and the Nursing and Midwifery Council (2018) *The Code.*

PROFESSIONAL

Department of Health and Welsh office (1999) *Mental* Health Act 1983 *Code of Practice.* Guidance from the professional organisations, such as *Consent in England and Wales* from the Royal College of Nursing (2022).

OTHER

A book discussing the legal and ethical principles of consent (Cornock, 2021) Employer policy on obtaining consent.
Consent forms and the associated guidance on their use.

There is no requirement for a healthcare practitioner to follow a particular policy or guidance if they do not believe that it is in the patient's best interests to do so. However, the healthcare practitioner needs to be able to justify their decision not to follow them and keep a clear record of how and why there has been a deviation from standard policy and/or guidance.

If something goes wrong and the healthcare practitioner has not followed an accepted policy or guidance that other healthcare practitioners do follow, there may be consequences for the healthcare practitioner. The healthcare practitioner's actions in not following the policy or guidance will be judged against the professional standard (professional standards are discussed in **Why is the professional standard important to a healthcare practitioner?** and **What is clinical negligence?**).

The consequences of a healthcare practitioner being seen as practising below the professional standard have been addressed in **Who can hold a healthcare practitioner professionally accountable?**

Q

Is it important for healthcare practitioners to record their decisions?

A

Yes. Very. Next question.

Sorry, you want a fuller answer. Oh, okay then.

Health records are a very important aspect of meeting a patient's healthcare needs. According to the Data Protection Act 2018, a health record *'consists of data concerning health and has been made by or on behalf of a health professional in connection with the diagnosis, care or treatment of the individual to whom the data relates'* (Section 205[1]).

Given that the purpose of a health record is to act as a complete record of the patient's interaction with healthcare services and healthcare practitioners, and thereby to ensure that they receive the care and treatment to meet their healthcare needs, its importance cannot be overstated.

One reason why healthcare practitioners should record their decisions is so that other practitioners can see what treatment is planned and why, and take over the patient's treatment if necessary, or to perform their part of the patient's care and treatment.

BRIEF ASIDE ON LEGAL DOCUMENTS

There is often talk of patient health records being legal documents and that because of this elevated status they need to be approached in a certain way. A legal document is any document that is needed in a legal matter. Therefore, any document could be a legal document, and no document is a legal document until it is required, for instance, in a clinical negligence claim.

There is an old adage that, if something a healthcare practitioner does is not written down, it hasn't happened. In relation to clinical practice, this is actually true from a legal and regulatory perspective. If a healthcare practitioner were to find that they had to defend their practice in a court or before a fitness to practise investigation, if there is no written record, an assumption will be made that the healthcare practitioner did not do what they claim they did because, if they had, they would have recorded it.

That is another reason why healthcare practitioners should record their decisions and their clinical practice activities.

A third reason for healthcare practitioners to record their clinical decisions is because it is part of their professional accountability. The statutory regulatory bodies require them to, and a failure to do so can be seen as not meeting the professional standard.

The Health and Care Professions Council's (2016) code of conduct states:

10.1 You must keep full, clear, and accurate records for everyone you care for, treat, or provide other services to.

10.2 You must complete all records promptly and as soon as possible after providing care, treatment or other services.

While the Nursing and Midwifery Council's (2018) code states that their registrants must:

10.1 complete records at the time or as soon as possible after an event, recording if the notes are written some time after the event

10.2 identify any risks or problems that have arisen and the steps taken to deal with them, so that colleagues who use the records have all the information they need

10.3 complete records accurately and without any falsification, taking immediate and appropriate action if you become aware that someone has not kept to these requirements

10.4 attribute any entries you make in any paper or electronic records to yourself, making sure they are clearly written, dated and timed, and do not include unnecessary abbreviations, jargon or speculation.

Q

Can healthcare practitioners treat themselves or their friends and relatives?

A

There is no legal prohibition on a healthcare practitioner treating themselves or their friends or family. The statutory regulatory body's codes of conduct do not prohibit it either. The Health and Care Professions Council's (HCPC's) code is silent on the matter while both the General Medical Council and the Nursing and Midwifery Council (NMC) codes merely say that whenever possible a registrant should avoid doing so.

The reason for not prohibiting it entirely is to cover an emergency situation where no other healthcare practitioner is available.

There are several reasons why it is inadvisable for healthcare practitioners to treat people that they '*have a close personal relationship*' with, to use the words of the General Medical Council (2013, at page 8).

A healthcare practitioner treating themselves, a friend or family member is unlikely to be truly independent as they will have a vested interest in the outcome of the treatment. That is not to say that the healthcare practitioner will be seeking to provide inappropriate care or treatment, just that they may want treatment to proceed in a certain direction.

Where the healthcare practitioner is treating themselves, it is very difficult for them to accurately assess their own symptoms, particularly if these include mental health symptoms.

There is also an issue of confidentiality, in that friends and family members of the healthcare practitioner may not want to share certain personal information with them that is pertinent to deciding the correct treatment option. By treating their friends and family members, it will mean the healthcare practitioner is privy to confidential information that they would not ordinarily have access to.

If the healthcare practitioner is treating themselves or their friends or family members independently of other healthcare provision, members of the healthcare team who normally care for that person will not be able to provide their input which may potentially mean that important information relevant to the patient's healthcare need is not taken into account. This is also true in reverse in that, by independently treating themselves or a friend or family member, the healthcare practitioner may inadvertently keep information from the patient's record that future healthcare practitioners would find useful when treating the patient.

Does conscientious objection absolve healthcare practitioners of their professional accountability?

There are times when a patient's treatment decision will conflict with a healthcare practitioner's beliefs.

In healthcare, conscientious objection is the mechanism whereby healthcare practitioners may exert their autonomy to practise in a way which reflects their own belief system, whether moral, ethical or religious.

Currently, there are two areas of healthcare where healthcare practitioners may exert a statutory right of conscientious objection. Section 4(1) of the Abortion Act 1967 states that *'no person shall be under any duty, whether by contract or by any statutory or other legal requirement, to participate in any treatment authorised by this Act to which he has a conscientious objection'*. This applies to healthcare practitioners working in England, Scotland and Wales. For healthcare practitioners working in Northern Ireland, Part 7 of The Abortion (Northern Ireland) Regulations 2020 has a similar provision.

Where a healthcare practitioner wishes to act upon a conscientious objection provision, they have to prove that they do indeed have a conscientious objection.

It is worth noting that the legal provisions regarding conscientious objection relating to termination of pregnancy do not mean that a healthcare practitioner can refuse to be involved with the care and treatment of a patient undergoing a termination of pregnancy. Both the Act and Regulations have provisions which require a healthcare practitioner to *'participate in treatment which is necessary to save the life, or to prevent grave permanent injury to the physical or mental health, of a pregnant woman'* (Abortion Act 1967 section 4(2) and The Abortion (Northern Ireland) Regulations 2020 section 12(3)), even if this means participating in a termination of pregnancy.

Additionally, it has been established in common law that the conscientious objection clause may only be invoked in relation to the actual act of the termination of pregnancy. Anything that comes before the actual act or after the pregnancy has ended will fall outside of the conscientious objection clause, and a healthcare practitioner will not be able to exclude themselves from these activities (Greater Glasgow Health Board v Doogan and another [2014], a case which had to decide if two midwives could object to being part of any aspect of abortion, including supervising or supporting staff participating in an abortion). There is also an obligation on a healthcare practitioner to ensure that, where they are unwilling to engage with a termination of pregnancy, they ensure that the patient is referred to someone who will take on the care and treatment of the patient. Until the patient is transferred to the care of that healthcare practitioner, they remain responsible for the patient's care and treatment.

The other area of healthcare practice where a healthcare practitioner may exert a statutory right of conscientious objection is in relation to the activities which are regulated by the Human Fertilisation and Embryology Act 1990, such as embryo research and those related to assisted conception (Human Fertilisation and Embryology Act 1990 section 38).

There have been attempts over the years to extend the areas for which a healthcare practitioner may exert a statutory right to conscientiously object to participate. The most recent of these was the Conscientious Objection (Medical Activities) Bill [HL] 2017–19, which was first introduced in the House of Lords on 28 June 2017 and progressed through to 23 March 2018. The Bill was intended to extend a healthcare practitioner's right to conscientious objection to the withdrawal of life-sustaining treatment as well as retaining the two areas previously discussed. It also intended to clarify what participation in the various activities meant.

The Bill did not become law because Parliament ended without the Bill going through all the necessary stages, and it has not been introduced in a subsequent session of Parliament. Therefore, at present, only the two areas discussed above are ones where a healthcare practitioner may exert a statutory right of conscientious objection.

Healthcare practitioners are professionally accountable for ensuring that all their patients receive the appropriate care and treatment, even where the healthcare practitioner is invoking their statutory right not to participate in certain areas of treatment due to a conscientious objection to that treatment. The onus is on the healthcare practitioner to care for and treat the patient until the care and treatment can be provided by another healthcare practitioner.

Q **What is patient safety and how do risk management, clinical governance and quality assurance contribute to it?**

A Patient safety, along with public protection, has been stated throughout his book as one of the reasons for the professional accountability of healthcare practitioners, for instance, see **Why are healthcare practitioners professionally accountable?** Indeed, patient safety has been linked to the professional status of healthcare practitioners and their regulation as whole.

It is probably too obvious to state but here goes anyway, patient safety is at the very core of healthcare practice and of the practice of healthcare practitioners, or should be!

For the World Health Organization (2022), *'the simplest definition of patient safety is the prevention of errors and adverse effects to patients associated with health care'*. While for NHS England (2022a), *'patient safety is the avoidance of unintended or unexpected harm to people during the provision of health care'*.

It seems rather unfortunate that the World Health Organisation still sees the need to hold a 'World Patient Safety Day' each year. Such days are used to draw attention to initiatives to improve patient safety. This would seem to suggest that patient safety cannot be taken for granted and that there is still work to be done to ensure that patients are safe when they receive healthcare.

That said, NHS England has a NHS Patient Safety Strategy, which according to its website *'describes how the NHS will continuously improve patient safety, building on the foundations of a safer culture and safer systems'* (NHS England, 2022b).

Maybe patient safety is not something that can be taken for granted after all, which is interesting given all the initiatives and polices that have been put in place over the years. Some of the more prominent of these initiatives include:

- Risk management
- Clinical governance
- Quality assurance

'Risk management is the systematic identification, assessment and evaluation of risk' according to Cottee and Harding (2008 at page 155). The aim of risk management is to identify potential or actual risks in healthcare and to minimise the effects of these through a variety of measures.

For Cottee and Harding (2008), *'risk management can be reactive (e.g. in response to a serious incident or a complaint), pro-active (e.g. establishment of a risk register or an assessment of national guidelines/reports) or preventative (e.g. ensuring adequate training and staffing levels)'* (at page 155).

Risk management is designed to spot a risk before it becomes an issue and put measures in place to prevent the risk materialising or to react to risks that have happened and prevent them reoccurring.

Clinical governance is noted by Chandraharan and Arulkumaran (2007) to be a *'framework through which NHS organisations are accountable for continuously improving the quality of their services and safeguarding high standards of care by creating an environment in which excellence in clinical care will flourish'* (at page 222).

While for Ellis (2019), *'clinical governance is a system whereby what nurses, and other care professionals, do in practice is subjected to scrutiny to ensure it is worthwhile, the correct policies and guidelines are in place, audit of practice is happening and money is spent wisely'* (at page 10).

Clinical governance is different to many policy initiatives in that it not only seeks to develop and maintain a high standard of care delivery, but it also seeks to constantly improve the delivery of care.

Quality assurance is probably the oldest of the three concepts presented here. Ellis and Whittington (1993) state that *'quality assurance is basically a simple idea. Standards are set for a product or service ... to apply the idea to health care, standards must be set for its delivery and everything must be managed to ensure that these standards are always met. Patients would therefore be assured that they would receive quality care'* (at page 1).

Through the setting of standards and the monitoring of the achievement of these standards, quality assurance sets the standard of the care that is delivered to patients. Essentially, the philosophy behind quality assurance is that, if you don't have a standard to achieve, how do you know what the quality threshold is and, more importantly, if you have met it or not? It is quality assurance that led to the setting of clinical standards throughout healthcare.

To answer the question how do risk management, clinical governance and quality assurance contribute to patient safety? They are all guiding principles for the delivery of healthcare. They either set a standard or framework which measures achievement against a quality threshold and look for ways to improve the quality or they identify where the quality threshold is at risk and seek ways to address that.

How does safeguarding relate to patient safety?

Safeguarding is associated with individuals who were seen as being vulnerable to abuse. However, Johnson and Boland (2019) maintain that *'the term 'vulnerable adult' was a term used in No Secrets to describe those adults who may need to be subject to safeguarding. However, in 2011, the Law commission recommended that this concept should no longer be used, as the label of vulnerability was not appropriate and could be 'stigmatising, dated, negative and disempowering'. The Care Act uses the term 'adult at risk' and also, at times, 'adult with care and support needs'* (at page 38).

The Care Act 2014 sets out various responsibilities and duties that exist in relation to adults at risk. While prior to the implementation of the Act in April 2015, various organisations had differing responsibilities and there could be confusion as to who was doing what, the Act clearly sets out the duties that exist and that an organisation must have a policy in place in relation to safeguarding which clearly sets out how it will fulfil its duty.

A useful definition of safeguarding is supplied by the Care Quality Commission (2022a) who state that *'safeguarding means protecting people's health, wellbeing and human rights, and enabling them to live free from harm, abuse and neglect. It's fundamental to high-quality health and social care'*.

The Care Quality commission goes on to note *'what safeguarding means for people who use care services'* and that *'safeguarding children and promoting their welfare includes:*

- *Protecting them from maltreatment or things that are bad for their health or development.*
- *Making sure they grow up in circumstances that allow safe and effective care.*

[While] *safeguarding adults includes:*

- *Protecting their rights to live in safety, free from abuse and neglect.*
- *People and organisations working together to prevent the risk of abuse or neglect, and to stop them from happening.*
- *Making sure people's wellbeing is promoted, taking their views, wishes, feelings and beliefs into account'* (Care Quality Commission, 2022a).

By having safeguarding measures in place, adults who are at risk should be identified and have their care and support needs met to minimise that risk. Thus, following the safeguarding principles is an extra layer of protection promoting patient safety during the time they are having their healthcare needs addressed.

See **How should a healthcare practitioner respond if they suspect a patient is being abused or neglected?** for actions a healthcare practitioner should take if they suspect a patient is at risk.

Q

How should a healthcare practitioner respond if they suspect a patient is being abused or neglected?

A

Unfortunately, there are many different forms of abuse that someone may be subjected to, including:

- Domestic violence
- Emotional abuse
- Financial abuse
- Neglect (including self-neglect)
- Organisational abuse
- Physical abuse

- Psychological abuse
- Sexual abuse
- Slavery

It is important to remember that anyone could be subject to abuse, not just those who may be considered vulnerable. Healthcare practitioners may encounter patients who are children or adults, including the elderly, competent or incompetent, who are being subject to one or more forms of abuse, or who may be abusing others.

Healthcare practitioners have a vital role in protecting patients from abuse and/or neglect. This is because they may have a patient in front of them who is being abused, have access to information that leads them to suspect abuse is occurring or witness behaviour that leads them to believe someone is being abused.

Abuse can sometimes continue to occur because no action has been taken against the abuser to protect the person being abused. Healthcare practitioners are not expected to stop a patient being abused by themselves, but they can report their concerns. Communication is key to identifying, preventing and stopping abuse. The more healthcare practitioners who do not report their concerns, the more likely that the abuse will continue.

When reporting concerns regarding suspected abuse, it is important to remember that patient information is confidential. Similarly, if a patient informs you that they are being abused, this is confidential.

As we saw when considering **When may confidential information be lawfully divulged?**, if the patient is an adult and competent, it is important to obtain their consent to divulge their confidential information to others. It is not possible to act in the best interests of a competent adult patient who will not consent to you divulging information about them. A competent adult is entitled to make their own decision even if this involves them suffering harm. As a healthcare practitioner, you should advise the patient of the options available to them and try to persuade them of options you consider to be in their best interests in a way that they can understand, but ultimately it is their decision. The only time you should go against a competent patient's wishes is where someone else is at risk of abuse, for example, children living with someone being abused, or where it is necessary in the public interest (as we saw in the question **When should confidential information be divulged?**).

If the patient is a child or an incompetent adult, you need to act in their best interests. This may involve reporting your concerns even where you cannot obtain consent to do so from the patient.

Where you do report your concerns, you should ensure this is to an appropriate authority/individual. You should only disclose the minimum amount of information that is necessary for the purpose of protecting the patient. You should also inform the patient of what you intend to do beforehand where this is possible.

Every clinical area should have a policy or procedure on how to deal with suspicions of abuse. There should be an individual identified who is a designated safeguarding or child protection lead, or a lead clinician to whom concerns can be reported. You should also approach the relevant person if you are unsure how to proceed.

If there is any doubt as to whether a specific patient is at risk of abuse, but you have a genuine reasonably held belief that they are, you should raise your concerns with the appropriate individual(s). As long as you are following the appropriate guidance and you only disclose information to relevant individual(s), your actions can be justified even if it turns out that there was no actual abuse occurring.

Q

Are healthcare practitioners allowed to have relationships with their patients?

A

The codes of conduct issued by the statutory regulatory bodies are a good starting point to address this question. While there is nothing that explicitly states that you cannot have a relationship in the NMC code, it does state that registrants must '*stay objective and have clear professional boundaries at all times with people in your care*' (Nursing and Midwifery Council, 2018 at paragraph 20.6).

The HCPC's code clearly states that registrants '*must keep your relationships with service users and carers professional*' (Health and Care Professions Council, 2016 at paragraph 1.7).

Regardless of the actual wording used in their respective codes, it is clear that the statutory regulatory bodies expect their registrants to be professional in their dealings with patients, and to have a clear boundary that recognises the healthcare relationship that exists and does not stray from the professional into the personal.

Several reasons could be put forward as to why personal relationships with patients are not a good idea.

The statutory regulatory bodies expect it of you is a rather good reason. Healthcare practitioners have been removed from the professional registers because of personal relationships with their patient(s).

When addressing **Are healthcare practitioners allowed to receive gifts from patients?**, it was stated that not only must a healthcare practitioner's practice be professional, but it must be seen to be professional. If a healthcare practitioner has a personal relationship with a patient, there is the possibility that some impropriety is occurring. While there may be no actual impropriety, the possibility that there could be means that the healthcare practitioner is not above suspicion and so not being seen to be professional, even if they are acting professionally.

Then there is the issue of the patient and whether the fact that they have a healthcare need that the healthcare practitioner is assisting them with means that they are vulnerable in some way. Relationships with vulnerable individuals raise the question of whether the vulnerable party has freely entered into the relationship or has been coerced in some way or is not able to exercise their choice not to be in the relationship.

In **Can healthcare practitioners treat themselves or their friends and relatives?**, treating relatives and friends was seen as being something to avoided whenever possible for a variety of reasons. All of those reasons apply to treating someone with whom the healthcare practitioner is in a relationship with.

The motives of the patient may also be questioned. For instance, has the patient entered into the relationship to obtain preferential treatment from the healthcare practitioner or to influence the healthcare practitioner into recommending a certain course of treatment?

It is not being suggested that the healthcare practitioner will consciously favour the patient with whom they have a relationship over their other patients, but how difficult might it be subconsciously to refuse your patient something they request if you are also in a personal relationship with them? On the other hand, if the relationship is not going well, the opposite may be true, and the healthcare practitioner may subconsciously withhold appropriate treatment from the patient with whom they are in a failing relationship.

For the reasons above, maintaining boundaries between the professional and the personal is the professional approach and is to be recommended.

Q / Can patients request a chaperone be present during examinations?

A   *'A chaperone is an impartial observer present during an intimate examination of a patient'* according to the Care Quality Commission (2022b).

Patients can request that a chaperone is present when they are examined by a healthcare practitioner; usually this is when an intimate examination is needed. Healthcare practitioners can also request that a chaperone is present if they have any concerns about the patient and/or their understanding of the examination.

While the healthcare practitioner is required to provide a chaperone when one is requested by a patient, or arrange for the examination to be rebooked if one is not available, a patient can refuse to have a chaperone present when it is a healthcare practitioner request. If the patient still refuses after the healthcare practitioner explains their reasoning for requesting a chaperone to be present, the healthcare practitioner needs to consider if the examination can wait until a colleague can undertake it or if they need to proceed without a chaperone.

Because chaperones need to be impartial, a relative or friend of the patient is not best placed to be a chaperone. Confidentiality issues could also be a concern. However, if the patient requests that a friend or relative is present, best practice would suggest that this should be in addition to the formal chaperone.

Chaperones should receive training for their role. Because they need training, it means that only certain individuals can act as chaperone and if one is not available, the steps described above should be followed.

The use of a chaperone should act as an additional reassurance for the patient, and/or the healthcare practitioner. It does not remove the need for healthcare practitioners to inform the patient of the reasons for an examination and how the examination will be undertaken. Any cultural or patient specific sensitives around examinations should be respected.

SUMMARY

- Clinical decision-making is a process whereby a healthcare practitioner utilises their competence and experience to provide safe and effective care for their patients.
- Where a patient wants to be fully involved in their healthcare, they should be encouraged to do so, receive the appropriate information and, where necessary, have the healthcare practitioner advocate for their participation. Where patients want limited involvement, this should be respected, and the patient assisted as much as is necessary.
- Shared decision-making is a process whereby a healthcare practitioner works with a patient to allow them to take as much of a role as they wish in making the decisions that will address their healthcare needs.
- Patients are only able to choose treatment from the options provided by a healthcare practitioner. They cannot demand a specific treatment. If they do not want the treatment that is being offered to them, they can refuse it, but they cannot replace it with another treatment that the healthcare practitioner is not willing to provide.
- Evidence-based practice is a systematic approach to using best available evidence to support clinical decision-making by healthcare practitioners and patients.
- Evidence-based practice is a means by which healthcare practitioners can demonstrate the rationale for their clinical decision-making.
- There are various forms of evidence that could be used to support clinical decision-making.
- Although hierarchies of evidence and their reliability exist, these have their limitations and it is the use that the evidence is put to that is more important than its place in a hierarchy.
- Although healthcare practitioners do not have to follow policies and guidance where it is not in their patient's best interests to do so, they may be taken as the professional standard and the healthcare practitioner needs to be able to justify their decision not to follow them.
- It is important for healthcare practitioners to record their clinical decisions and their clinical activities to ensure that patients receive the correct care and treatment; to meet their professional accountability; and because a failure to do so could be seen as not meeting the professional standard.
- Healthcare practitioners should avoid treating themselves or their friends or family members because they may not have all the relevant information on which to base treatment decisions; they may have a vested interest in pursuing certain treatment options over other treatments; it raises issues in relation to confidentiality; and it may prevent healthcare practitioners in the future from being aware of the clinical episode and treatment provided and so hinder the patient's future healthcare needs.

- Healthcare practitioners are professionally accountable for ensuring that all their patients receive the appropriate care and treatment, even where the healthcare practitioner is invoking their statutory right not to participate in certain areas of treatment due to a conscientious objection to that treatment. The onus is on the healthcare practitioner to care for and treat their patient until the care and treatment can be provided by another healthcare practitioner.
- Risk management, clinical governance and quality assurance are all guiding principles for the delivery of healthcare and either set a standard or framework which measures achievement against a quality threshold and look for ways to improve the quality or they identify where the quality threshold is at risk of being missed and seek ways to address that.
- Safeguarding principles are an extra layer of protection promoting patient safety during the time they are having their healthcare needs addressed.
- A healthcare practitioner should report any concerns they have regarding the abuse or neglect of a patient according to local policy.
- Healthcare practitioners should be advised that they should maintain a boundary between their personal and professional lives and avoid personal relationships with their patients.
- Both patients and healthcare practitioners can request that a chaperone is present during clinical examinations. If the patient makes the request, this should be arranged or the examination postponed until a chaperone is available.

REFERENCES

Abortion Act 1967.

Birrell Ivory, S. (2021) *Becoming a Critical Thinker*. Oxford University Press: Oxford.

Care Act 2014.

Care Quality Commission (2022a) *Safeguarding People*. Available at: https://www.cqc.or-g.uk/what-we-do/how-we-do-our-job/safeguarding-people

Care Quality Commission (2022b) *GP Mythbuster 15: Chaperones*. Available at: https://www.cqc.org.uk/guidance-providers/gps/gp-mythbuster-15-chaperones

Chandraharan, E. and Arulkumaran, S. (2007) 'Clinical governance', *Obstetrics, Gynaecology and Reproductive Medicine*, 17(7): 222–224.

Children Act 1989.

Conscientious Objection (Medical Activities) Bill [HL] 2017-19.

Cornock, M. (2021) *Key Questions in Healthcare Law and Ethics*. SAGE: London.

Cottee, C. and Harding, K. (2008) 'Risk management in obstetrics', *Obstetrics, Gynaecology and Reproductive Medicine*, 18(6): 155–162.

Data Protection Act 2018.

Department of Health and Welsh Office (1999) *Mental Health Act 1983 Code of Practice*. The Stationery Office: London.

Ellis, P. (2019) *Evidence-Based Practice in Nursing* (4th edition). SAGE: London.

Ellis, R. and Whittington, D. (1993) *Quality Assurance in Health Care*. Edward Arnold: London.

General Medical Council (2013) *Good Medical Practice*. General Medical Council: London.

Gillick v West Norfolk and Wisbech Area Health Authority and another [1985] 3 ALL ER 402.

Gray, J. (1997) *Evidence-Based Healthcare*. Churchill Livingstone: Edinburgh.

Greater Glasgow Health Board (Appellant) v Doogan and another (Respondents) (Scotland) [2014] UKSC 68.

Health and Care Professions Council (2016) *Standards of Conduct, Performance and Ethics*. Health and Care Professions Council: London.

Johnson, K. and Boland, B. (2019) 'Adult safeguarding under the Care Act 2014', *British Journal of Psychiatry Bulletin*, 43: 38–42.

Lamont, T. (2021) *Making Research Matter*. Policy Press: Bristol.

Mental Capacity Act 2005.

Montgomery v Lanarkshire Health Board [2015] UKSC 11.

National Institute for Health and Care Excellence (NICE) (2022) *Developing NICE Guidelines: The Manual. Process and Methods (PMG20)*. Available at: www.nice.org.uk/process/pmg20/chapter/glossary

NHS England (2022a) *Patient Safety*. Available at: https://www.england.nhs.uk/patient-safety/

NHS England (2022b) *The NHS Patient Safety Strategy*. Available at: https://www.england.nhs.uk/patient-safety/the-nhs-patient-safety-strategy/

Nursing and Midwifery Council (2018) *The Code*. Nursing and Midwifery Council: London.

Royal College of Nursing (2022) *Consent in England and Wales*. Available at: https://www.rcn.org.uk/clinical-topics/consent/consent-in-england-and-wales

Sackett, D., Rosenberg, W., Gray, J., Haynes, R. and Richardson, W. (1996) 'Evidence based medicine: What it is and what it isn't', *British Medical Journal*, 312(7023): 71–72.

Secretary of State for Health (2000) *The NHS Plan: A Plan for Investment, a Plan for Reform Cm 4818-I*. The Stationery Office: London.

Standing, M. (2005) 'Perceptions of clinical decision-making on a developmental journey from student to staff nurse'. PhD thesis, Canterbury, University of Kent, in Standing, M. (ed) (2010) Clinical Judgement and Decision-Making. Open University Press: Maidenhead.

The Abortion (Northern Ireland) Regulations 2020 (SI 2020/345).

Thompson, A. (2007) 'The meaning of patient invent and participation in health care consultations: A taxonomy', *Social Science and Medicine*, 64(6): 1297–1310.

Wilkinson, C. (ed) (2007) *Professional Perspectives in Health Care*. Palgrave: Basingstoke.

World Health Organization (2022) *Patient Safety*. Available at: https://www.who.int/europe/health-topics/patient-safety#tab=tab_1

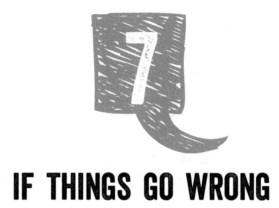

IF THINGS GO WRONG

Chapter 7 discusses the healthcare practitioner's professional accountability from the perspective of things going wrong during the delivery of healthcare or where there is a suspicion that they are going to go wrong.

The chapter starts by looking at ways in which a healthcare practitioner can raise their concerns and how mistakes can be used positively, before examining the potential ways a healthcare practitioner may be involved if something goes wrong.

Explaining events that have not gone to plan to patients is considered along with the duty of candour, as well as noting whether it is appropriate to say sorry.

Chapter 7 also considers healthcare practitioners who expand their area of competence and those who act outside of their clinical environment, to examine if this changes their professional accountability.

QUESTIONS COVERED IN CHAPTER 7

- How might a healthcare practitioner be involved if something goes wrong?
- Do healthcare practitioners have to challenge poor practice?
- How should a healthcare practitioner raise their concerns about systems and resources?
- Is whistleblowing different to raising a concern?
- How can healthcare practitioners benefit from mistakes?
- Why is there a duty of candour?
- Is the professional duty of candour different to the duty of candour?
- Are there any problems with saying sorry to patients?
- How should complaints be approached?
- What happens at a Coroner's Inquest?
- What is clinical negligence?
- Are there any special considerations in the duty of care or standard of care?

- What is a fitness to practise investigation?
- Can a healthcare practitioner be investigated for personal as well as professional issues?
- What sanctions can be imposed by a statutory regulatory body?
- What should you do if, despite all your professional efforts, something does go wrong in your practice?

Q
A

How might a healthcare practitioner be involved if something goes wrong?

There are times in healthcare practice when things do not go to plan. The right patient does not receive the right treatment at the right time. Or, if they do, an unexpected or unintended event occurs. When these events do occur, they can have both serious and permanent consequences for the patients affected.

There are two main ways in which a healthcare practitioner may be involved in healthcare going wrong. The first is before the event, where the healthcare practitioner may be highlighting potential areas of concern, and the second is after the event, where the healthcare practitioner will be involved in the potential consequences of the concern actually happening. Regardless of whether the healthcare practitioner is involved before or after the event, certain processes will need to be followed.

These processes relate to the categories of professional accountability that were explored in **Who can hold a healthcare practitioner professionally accountable?** In the rest of this answer, the processes are just discussed alphabetically rather than in order of severity of outcome for the healthcare practitioner or any other order of seriousness.

- Civil action
Patients are able to make a claim against healthcare practitioners for wrongdoing that they say the healthcare practitioner has done. This is commonly known as the patient suing the healthcare practitioner.

The two main reasons for the patient to sue their healthcare practitioner are because they believe the healthcare practitioner has acted negligently or because the healthcare practitioner has breached their confidentiality.

Negligence is discussed in **What is clinical negligence?** while breach of confidence is considered in **What happens if a healthcare practitioner breaches a patient's confidentiality?**

- Complaints, which are explored in **How should complaints be approached?**

- Coroner's Inquests and, in Scotland, Fatal Accident Inquiries, which are reviewed in **What happens at a Coroner's Inquest?**

- Criminal investigations
This is a very specialised area and one that is outside the scope of this book. For the purposes of this answer, the following is a very brief overview.

Where it is suspected that a crime has been committed, the police will undertake a criminal investigation. If their investigation leads them to believe that there is enough evidence to charge the healthcare practitioner with a specific crime(s), they will contact the Crown Prosecution Service who will decide whether to prosecute the healthcare practitioner or not. If the healthcare practitioner is found guilty, the possible sentences include a fine, community order or custodial order (imprisonment). Any of these could be suspended meaning that they will not be imposed unless the person breaks the terms of the suspension.

If you are ever the subject of a police investigation, make sure that you seek representation by a solicitor who can advise you.

- Employer disciplinary processes, which are reviewed in **Who can hold a healthcare practitioner professionally accountable?**

- Inquiries, which are discussed in **What is being regulated?**

- Raising concerns

There are two main areas that a healthcare practitioner may want to raise a concern about: colleagues, and systems and resources.

Raising a concern in relation to a colleague(s) is discussed in **If I have concerns about a colleague what should I do?**

Raising a concern about a system issue or resources is explored in **How should a healthcare practitioner raise their concerns about systems and resources?**

- Statutory regulatory body investigations about fitness to practise, which are considered in **What is a fitness to practise investigation?**

- University fitness to practise investigations, which are reviewed in **Are student healthcare practitioners professionally accountable?**

- Whistleblowing, discussed in **Is whistleblowing different to raising a concern?**

Q

Do healthcare practitioners have to challenge poor practice?

A

Poor practice can be defined as anything that results in the patient receiving care that falls below the accepted standard. Poor practice can be related to the healthcare practitioner(s) delivering the care to the patient, or it can be related to the systems and resources that the healthcare practitioner uses.

When patients are subject to poor practice, they are receiving care that falls below the accepted standard, that is, they are receiving substandard care. If a patient is not receiving the care and treatment they need to meet their healthcare needs, they are likely to suffer as a result. This suffering could be a delay in their recovery or other harm.

Healthcare practitioners do not practise to see their patients suffer; therefore, it could be expected that all healthcare practitioners would want to challenge each and every instance of poor practice that they witness.

It is part of the healthcare practitioner's professional accountability as discussed in **Why are healthcare practitioners professionally accountable?** that they maintain and promote patient safety as part of their professional mandate. It is in the healthcare practitioner's, and their profession's, interest that patient safety is seen to be being promoted because it helps to ensure the profession's continued existence without additional regulatory oversight.

Many healthcare practitioners will find that their contract of employment and/or their roles and responsibilities as set out in a job description will have a clause that requires them to raise concerns they have about things that could affect patient safety.

As has been discussed in several of the questions and answers in this book, patient safety is a fundamental aspect of professions and professional accountability and that it is one of the defining reasons for the regulation of healthcare practitioners. Thus, this is why the statutory regulatory bodies require their registrants to challenge instances of poor practice when they occur.

The Health and Care Professions Council (2016) have a section in their code entitled 'Report concerns about safety' which clearly sets out its expectations that its registrants will 'report any concerns about the safety or well-being of service users promptly and appropriately' (at paragraph 7.1). Not only this, but the Health and Care Professions Council (2016) require their registrants to go beyond reporting their own concerns to 'support and encourage others to report concerns and not prevent anyone from raising concerns' (at paragraph 7.2). Additionally, for those healthcare practitioners who are on the registers of the Health and Care Professions Council, their obligation does not end with the reporting of their concerns and/or supporting and encouraging other healthcare practitioners to do the same, because the Health and Care Professions Council (2016) require them to 'follow up concerns you have reported and, if necessary, escalate them' (at paragraph 7.3).

Similarly, the Nursing and Midwifery Council (2018) state that registrants must 'act without delay if you believe that there is a risk to patient safety or public protection' (at paragraph 16) and to achieve this the registrant will need to 'raise and, if necessary, escalate any concerns you may have about patient or public safety, or the level of care people are receiving in your workplace or any other health and care setting' (at paragraph 16.1).

From their codes of conduct, there can be little doubt that the statutory regulatory bodies expect their registrants to challenge poor practice by reporting their concerns.

So do healthcare practitioners have to challenge poor practice? Yes, because their profession requires them to as part of their upholding of the professional standard; because as healthcare practitioners their raison d'etre is to promote patient safety; and it is a requirement of their professional accountability as outlined in their statutory regulatory body code of conduct.

Q How should a healthcare practitioner raise their concerns about systems and resources?

A This answer is concerned with occasions when healthcare practitioners have a concern regarding a system or process or resources rather than when their concern is in relation to fellow healthcare practitioner(s). For concerns about healthcare practitioner(s) see **If I have concerns about a colleague what should I do?**

The reasons that a healthcare practitioner may have a concern in relation to systems and resources include:

- Workloads – for example, where the healthcare practitioner does not consider that there is an adequate number of staff present to meet the needs of the patients in the clinical area.
- Skill mix – where there may be an adequate number of staff present in the clinical area, but the healthcare practitioner does not consider that the proportion of trained to untrained, or registered to unregistered, or qualified to student means that the roles that need to be undertaken by the team can be fulfilled.
- Lack of resources – which may be related to an insufficient amount of vital equipment being present, or a lack of supplies necessary to meet the needs of the patients.

It is not easy to raise a concern because of a worry about what will happen to you or because you may be 'causing trouble' for others, or that your concern is unfounded, but knowing that it is a means of protecting patients from potential harm and a requirement of satisfying your professional accountability may be of help to those healthcare practitioners who have concerns. Additionally, it may be that no-one else is aware of the issue behind the concern that the healthcare practitioner has and so by raising it, they are bringing it to the attention of those who can act upon it and resolve it.

To those healthcare practitioners who do not think that they should report a concern they have, the question they need to answer is **what will happen if the situating continues because it is not reported?**

It may be better to report a concern that is already known about and being addressed than to not raise a concern and see a patient suffer because of it. Additionally, the earlier a concern is raised the lower the risk that it will escalate and become a more major issue.

There are two types of concern that the healthcare practitioner may wish to raise: those that pose an immediate threat to patient safety and those that do not pose an immediate risk but will become a risk if they are not addressed.

There are many sources of support and guidance in relation to raising a concern; the statutory regulatory bodies provide information on the duty to raise a concern and how this should be undertaken; the professional support bodies (see **What is the association between professional support organisations, accountability and being a professional?** for discussion on the role of professional support organisations) produce guidance on raising a concern and some provide support to their members when raising a concern; employers will have a policy on raising concerns which should detail the process to be followed and may include contact details for support in raising a concern, for instance, from the Human Resources department; for student healthcare practitioners, universities will have a policy on how to raise a concern and who it should be raised with.

There are some general principles to follow when raising a concern:

- If the risk is immediate, the concern should be raised urgently.
- Wherever possible, follow the local policy for raising a concern.
- In many instances, there will be a route for a concern to be raised informally (where there is no immediate risk).
- If you can, seek support to raise your concern. This could be from a professional support organisation, a trade union, a colleague, mentor, supervisor or friend.
- If you are unsure of where to raise the concern, the best course of action is to discuss it with your line manager who either should be able to act upon it, or will know how to take it further so that the appropriate action can be taken.
- When raising the concern, stick to the facts and be objective about what the concern is and why it is being raised and, if appropriate, what you think needs to happen to resolve it.
- Respect patient confidentiality when raising the concern.
- Keep a record of the concern you raised, your reason for raising it, who you raised it with, the method by which you raised it (for instance, in person, by telephone or email etc.) and the date and time that you raised it.
- Know that once you have raised a concern, no one can say that they were not aware of the issue.
- You may need to follow up your concern if there is no apparent resolution of the issue.

Is whistleblowing different to raising a concern?

It should be noted that strictly speaking whistleblowing can refer to raising a concern either within an organisation or externally to the organisation.

However, raising a concern, as discussed in **If I have concerns about a colleague what should I do?** and **How should a healthcare practitioner raise their concerns about systems and resources?**, is generally associated with highlighting the issue within an organisation.

Sometimes concerns are not acted upon adequately, and the risk that caused the concern still exists or has even escalated, and the healthcare practitioner has exhausted all the local routes to having the concern addressed and so has to go externally to their organisation to have their concern addressed. This is what is more commonly referred to as whistleblowing, and the rest of this answer will assume that whistleblowing refers to when the concern is being raised externally.

As with raising a concern, there are various sources of guidance and support when a healthcare practitioner is considering whistleblowing, and it would be best practice to consult these before actually whistleblowing.

There is legal protection in place for whistleblowers, and this is through the Public Interest Disclosure Act 1998. The legal protections should mean that a healthcare practitioner is not treated unfairly or to suffer a detriment in their employment because of their whistleblowing.

In order to have the protection afforded to whistleblowers, the healthcare practitioner has to make what is known as a *'protected disclosure'* (section 43A Public Interest Disclosure Act 1998).

An act of whistleblowing will be a protected disclosure if it meets the conditions set out in sections 43B to 43L of the Public Interest Disclosure Act 1998. These conditions include that the disclosure:

- Is made in good faith
- Is not made for financial gain
- Is made in the reasonable belief of the whistleblower that certain wrongdoings either have occurred or are likely to occur; these include *'that the health or safety of any individual has been, is being or is likely to be endangered'* (section 43B(d))
- Is made in the public interest
- Is made to the employer or, where the whistleblower believes they would suffer a detriment if they made the disclosure to their employer, to one or more prescribed persons

It is vital to note that a whistleblower may only make their disclosure to their employer or a prescribed person; this has to be someone or an organisation that can act on the issue which is causing the concern.

Prescribed persons include:

- Legal advisers
- Ministers of the Crown
- Statutory regulatory bodies
- Care Quality Commission

The type of issue which may give rise to whistleblowing includes anything that is or may cause harm to patients, including staffing levels, lack or resources or an inappropriate skill mix, safeguarding issues or the actions of colleagues.

It can be seen from the above that whistleblowing to a newspaper, whether for payment or not, would not satisfy the requirements under the Public Interest Disclosure Act 1998, and so the whistleblower would not have the protections afforded by the Act.

Finally, it is very important not to breach patient confidentiality when whistleblowing.

Q **How can healthcare practitioners benefit from mistakes?**

A Mistakes are not something that a healthcare practitioner wants to make. It implies that they did something that they did not mean to do, or the outcome was not what they intended to happen. Therefore, asking how a healthcare practitioner can benefit from doing something they didn't intend or resulted in unintended consequences may seem rather perverse. However, bear with this for a moment.

Mistakes that result in harm to patients are bad, but they happen. They can be dealt with at the time and sometimes they can be rectified and at others the patient suffers, and this cannot be resolved. Sometimes patients die as a result of a mistake by a healthcare practitioner. Indeed, there is an old adage about healthcare practitioners burying their mistakes. This is not meant to be facile or to lessen the effect of mistakes or to fail to acknowledge the suffering that can occur for the patient or the distress for the healthcare practitioner. The point that is being made is that however much we wish it were otherwise mistakes do and will happen during the delivery of healthcare and patients will suffer as a consequence of these mistakes, but benefits can arise as result of a mistake.

There is a quotation which is attributed to Winston Churchill but is said to be a misquotation, whether intentional or not, of George Santayana: *those who fail to learn from history are condemned to repeat it*. In the context of mistakes in healthcare, this can be taken as healthcare practitioners have to learn from their mistakes or they will repeat them.

Learning from mistakes is not easy; however, it is essential. As Alan Milburn said when Secretary of State for Health in 2000 '*too often in the past we have witnessed tragedies which could have been avoided had the lessons of past experience been properly learned*' (Department of Health, 2000 at page v).

Clinical governance, which is discussed in **What is patient safety and how do risk management, clinical governance and quality assurance contribute to it?,** can be said to be an organisation-level approach to learning from mistakes. Through its commitment to quality improvement, it requires a review of where mistakes have occurred so that improvements can be made that will reduce the risk of them occurring in the future.

Such is the need to learn from mistakes that an expert group was established to report on how this could be accomplished in the National Health Service. The report of this expert group, *An organisation with a memory* (Department of Health, 2000), resulted in a number of recommendations that would enable or enhance opportunities to learn from mistakes, for instance, the reporting of mistakes, known as adverse events in the report, on a national basis so that an issue in one part of the National Health Service could result in lessons being learnt in another part. There was also a recommendation that mistakes that do not result in an adverse event because it was averted at the last moment or because it did not fully materialise, known as a near miss in the report, should also be reported. This is because what is a near miss today could have a tragic consequence tomorrow and because learning from a mistake that did not result in a patient suffering could be easier for the healthcare practitioners involved than one where a patient did suffer.

Healthcare practitioners can benefit from mistakes, whether made by them or others, by learning from them, either at an individual level or at the level of the organisation, and apply what they have learnt so that the mistake is not repeated. By learning from mistakes and adjusting their practice in the light of that learning, healthcare practitioners demonstrate how their professional accountability is used to ensure patient safety.

Q Why is there a duty of candour?

A The duty of candour can be directly linked to the Mid Staffordshire scandal. Campbell (2013) states that *'between 400 and 1,200 patients died as a result of poor care over the 50 months between January 2005 and March 2009 at Stafford hospital, a small district general hospital in Staffordshire'*.

A public inquiry was commissioned in June 2010 and published its findings in a report in February 2013. Commonly known as the Francis Inquiry, after its Chair, there were 290 recommendations made by the Inquiry.

One failing highlighted by the Francis Inquiry was a culture that sought to present a positive image, as Stafford Hospital belonged to the Mid Staffordshire NHS Hospital Trust (which is the reason the scandal has been called the Mid Staffordshire scandal) was seeking to achieve foundation trust status. It was noted that a culture of fear was present throughout the Trust with regard to raising failings.

In order to counter this in the future, the report of the Francis Inquiry stated that *'the common culture of caring requires a displacement of a culture of fear with a culture of openness, honesty and transparency, where the only fear is the failure to uphold the fundamental standards and the caring culture'* (at paragraph 1.180 of the Mid Staffordshire NHS Foundation Trust Public Inquiry Executive Summary (2013).

Further that this had to be instilled through the National Health Service and that this would require three characteristics:

Openness: enabling concerns to be raised and disclosed freely without fear, and for questions to be answered;

Transparency: allowing true information about performance and outcomes to be shared with staff, patients and the public;

Candour: ensuring that patients harmed by a healthcare service are informed of the fact and that an appropriate remedy is offered (at paragraph 1.176 of the Mid Staffordshire NHS Foundation Trust Public Inquiry Executive Summary, 2013).

In order to change the culture, 12 of the 290 recommendations (numbers 173–184) made by the Francis Inquiry were concerned with the principles of openness, transparency and candour. The Government published its response to the Francis Inquiry report in January 2014 (Department of Health, 2014). Not all the recommendations made by the Francis Inquiry were adopted by the Government.

One of the recommendations of the Francis Inquiry that was adopted was in relation to a duty of candour, as stated in the response document *'we are introducing a statutory duty of candour on all heath providers, making it a requirement for them to be open and honest where there have been failings in care'* (Department of Health, 2014 at page 10).

The duty of candour is contained within regulation 20 of The Health and Social Care Act 2008 (Regulated Activities) Regulations 2014.

Regulation 20 is titled the *'duty of candour'*, and regulation 20(1) states that *'a health service body must act in an open and transparent way with relevant persons in relation to care and treatment provided to service users in carrying on a regulated activity'*. There are various requirements within the regulation as to how the duty of candour must be performed. These include that patients must be informed of incidents as soon as is practical after the event; that all the known facts be given; support must be given to individuals affected by the incident; an apology must be given; and that a record is kept of the incident.

Q

A

Is the professional duty of candour different to the duty of candour?

When discussing **Why is there a duty of candour?**, the duty of candour which arose as a result of the Francis Inquiry was raised. This is often known as the statutory duty of candour because the legal requirement to perform the duty arises in regulation 20 of The Health and Social Care Act 2008 (Regulated Activities) Regulations 2014.

The professional duty of candour is different to the statutory duty of candour because the statutory duty of candour only applies to service providers and not to individual healthcare practitioners. Because of this, the Chief Executives of the statutory regulatory bodies issued a joint statement in October 2014 entitled *Openness and honesty – the professional duty of candour* (Chief Executives of statutory regulators of healthcare professionals, 2014).

The joint statement had the effect of imposing a duty of candour on the registrants of the statutory regulatory bodies; they called this the professional duty of candour to differentiate it from the statutory duty of candour.

The professional duty of candour is:

Every healthcare professional must be open and honest with patients when something goes wrong with their treatment or care which causes, or has the potential to cause, harm or distress.

This means that healthcare professionals must:

- tell the patient (or, where appropriate, the patient's advocate, carer or family) when something has gone wrong;
- apologise to the patient (or, where appropriate, the patient's advocate, carer or family);

- offer an appropriate remedy or support to put matters right (if possible); and
- explain fully to the patient (or, where appropriate, the patient's advocate, carer or family) the short and long term effects of what has happened (Chief Executives of statutory regulators of healthcare professionals, 2014).

Interestingly, all the Chief Executives of the statutory regulatory bodies signed the joint statement apart from the Chief Executive of the Health and Care Professions Council. However, all healthcare practitioners who are registrants with one of the statutory bodies have the professional duty of candour as it has been incorporated into the various codes of conduct. For registrants of the Health and Care Professions Council, the duty is in paragraph 8.1 which states:

You must be open and honest when something has gone wrong with the care, treatment or other services that you provide by:

- informing service users or, where appropriate, their carers, that something has gone wrong;
- apologising;
- taking action to put matters right if possible; and
- making sure that service users or, where appropriate, their carers, receive a full and prompt explanation of what has happened and any likely effects. (Health and Care Professions Council, 2016)

For registrants of the Nursing and Midwifery Council, the duty arises in paragraph 14 of 'The Code' which states:

Be open and candid with all service users about all aspects of care and treatment, including when any mistakes or harm have taken place

To achieve this, you must:

14.1 act immediately to put right the situation if someone has suffered actual harm for any reason or an incident has happened which had the potential for harm.

14.2 explain fully and promptly what has happened, including the likely effects, and apologise to the person affected and, where appropriate, their advocate, family or carers

14.3 document all these events formally and take further action (escalate) if appropriate so they can be dealt with quickly. (Nursing and Midwifery Council, 2018)

Q

Are there any problems with saying sorry to patients?

A

There is a belief among healthcare practitioners that you should never say sorry, or indeed apologise in any way, to a patient if a mistake or incident has occurred which involves them, even, or especially, if they have suffered any harm. Just so we all know what we mean by saying sorry or apologising, Regulation 20(7) of The Health and Social Care Act 2008 (Regulated Activities) Regulations 2014 defines an apology as *'an expression of sorrow or regret in respect of a notifiable safety incident'*.

When asked why healthcare practitioners should not apologise to their patients, most healthcare practitioners who agree that it should not be done say that it is because if you apologise to a patient you are admitting liability for the mistake or incident.

There is a small fallacy behind this line of reasoning and some illogical thinking. That is, if the healthcare practitioner was involved in the mistake or incident, they will have liability for their part anyway, and their liability does not increase because they have apologised. If the healthcare practitioner was not involved in the mistake or incident, liability cannot be placed on them merely because they have expressed their regret to the patient that the mistake or incident happened.

Saying sorry is actually a requirement of both the statutory and professional duties of candour (as explored in **Why is there a duty of candour?** and **Is the professional duty of candour different to the duty of candour?**), so both healthcare organisations and healthcare practitioners are obliged to say sorry to patients.

Apart from the legal and professional obligation to say sorry to patients, there are other reasons why saying sorry is good practice for healthcare practitioners. One reason is that it represents best practice and that it allows a patient to know that although a mistake has occurred, it has been acknowledged, and steps will be taken to resolve any issues.

So that there is no excuse to avoid saying sorry to patients and to clarify the position regarding liability for those who healthcare practitioners do fulfil their obligation to apologise, Section 2 of the Compensation Act 2006 states *'an apology, an offer of treatment or other redress, shall not of itself amount to an admission of negligence or breach of statutory duty'*. In short, merely saying sorry will not impose a liability where none previously existed or increase the liability that a healthcare practitioner would otherwise face.

Q

How should complaints be approached?

A

'I have just received a complaint about you' are not words that any healthcare practitioner wants to hear. A complaint is an expression of dissatisfaction with an aspect of the care that the patient has received.

Complaints can be directed at individual healthcare practitioners or about a team or a service. They can be informal or formal. The difference between the two being that a formal complaint requires a formal response, while an informal complaint may be resolved by speaking with the complainant and agreeing a course of action.

For patients who want to complain about an aspect of care within the National Health Service, there is specific guidance that explains how to complain as well as what they can expect in response to their complaint including the time limits for the various stages that are used to deal with the patient's complaint. Each of the four nations of the United Kingdom has their own complaints' policy and guidance.

Complaints can be made for a variety of reasons including that the patient wants:

- To alert someone to poor practice
- Information about an event
- Someone to say sorry
- To prevent the incident happening to other patients
- To blame someone for what happened

NHS organisations must have a complaints policy in place, and other healthcare service providers will generally do so. These will detail the steps that anyone dealing with a complaint has to perform. However, it is likely that most organisations will have a specific department or individual(s) who will deal with all formal complaints. The role of the healthcare practitioner who receives a complaint is to ensure that it is passed to the correct individual to deal with it on their behalf.

As part of the complaints process, healthcare practitioners may be asked to make a statement in response to the patient's complaint. If asked to make a statement, you may need to refer to the patient's health record. You should ensure that any statement you make is factual and addresses the points that the patient raises as part of their complaint. If there are any aspects of the complaint that you are unable to address, you should note these in your statement.

It is good practice to discuss the actual complaint with your colleagues to obtain different perspectives on the complaint and to seek support when writing a statement.

When responding to a complaint it is permissible to offer an apology, and this does not indicate any liability (see **Are there any problems with saying sorry to patients?**).

Although they are not necessarily welcomed, complaints can be approached as a part of the quality assurance process and as a learning opportunity, as discussed in **How can healthcare practitioners benefit from mistakes?**

Q What happens at a Coroner's Inquest?

A Healthcare practitioners may be called upon to give a written statement and/or to attend a Coroner's Inquest into the death of a patient in a healthcare setting.

The purpose of a Coroner's Inquest is to determine who the deceased person is and when, where and how they died. Scotland does not have a Coroner's Inquest as in the rest of the United Kingdom; there is a system of Fatal Accident Inquiries which investigate certain types of death.

Coroners are not judges but independent judicial officers, and work within a specified district. Their role and duties are contained within legislation such as the Coroners Rules 1984 and the Coroners Act 1988.

Coroners have the power to act when a body is within their district, and there is a reasonable suspicion of unnatural death, sudden death, violent death or the cause of death is unknown. They are also empowered to act when deaths occur in prisons.

When notified of a death, the coroner will decide if a death certificate can be issued, in which case the case will be closed, or if an autopsy or post-mortem examination is needed to determine the cause of death and/or if an inquest is needed.

Coroners are assisted by Coroners Officers. Coroners Officers can arrange for the removal of the body and may make enquiries relating to the cause of death, and interview witnesses and take their statements. They also arrange the hearing and can summon a jury and witnesses to attend.

Not all Coroners Inquests involve a jury; generally, juries are only present when the death occurred in a prison or where the health and safety of the public may be affected by the circumstances of the death being investigated.

A Coroner's Inquest is different to cases heard in the criminal and civil courts. Coroners decide which witnesses to call, and the process is inquisitorial and not adversarial. This means that it is not based on one side trying to prove their case against another side but is centred on trying to determine a set of facts to reach a conclusion on the circumstances of the deceased's death.

When the death has occurred in a healthcare setting, the normal process is for the coroner to request a list of witnesses and statements from those healthcare practitioners identified as witnesses through the NHS Trust or other organisation rather than contacting the healthcare practitioner directly.

Generally, a statement is required of a witness, and this will be read as part of the actual Coroner's Inquest. If a healthcare practitioner is asked to prepare a statement, it is permissible for the NHS Trust to prepare a draft or to offer assistance with the writing of the statement.

If a healthcare practitioner is required to give evidence in person, this will be given under oath or affirmation. The healthcare practitioner will be questioned directly by the coroner although other interested parties may also be permitted to question the witness. The coroner has the power and discretion to disallow questions which they deem are improper, and this means that the healthcare practitioner would not have to answer them.

There are no closing statements given by lawyers or the coroner. The coroner gives the verdict themselves unless it is one of the occasions when they are sitting with a jury. Verdicts available to a coroner, or the jury, include:

- Accident
- Industrial disease
- Misadventure
- Natural causes

- Neglect
- Open – where there is insufficient evidence to use one of the other verdicts
- Suicide
- Unlawful killing
- Unnatural causes

Coroners do not deal with blame, and verdicts must not identify an individual who has criminal or civil liability for the death. They are able to report the death to another authority, who must respond, if in the coroner's opinion action is needed to prevent other deaths in similar circumstances.

Q

A

What is clinical negligence?

Negligence is a specific form of tort, where a civil action is brought by one individual against another because they believe they have stuffed harm as a result of the other's actions. Bringing a civil action means that the person who brings the case, the claimant, has to prove their case against the person they are suing, the defendant, on the balance of probabilities, which means that one side's argument is believed more than the other's.

An everyday definition of the term negligence would be when a person is careless or reckless in undertaking a task that results in some measurable harm to another person.

Negligence as a legal action first arose in 1932 in the Donoghue case.

The reason that this case is said to have established the modern form of negligence is because it was in this case that it was held a duty of care was deemed to exist between two parties, even if there is no contractual relationship between them, and the parties are required to take due care in their dealings with each other. The establishment of a duty between individuals and the need to act in a certain way towards each other is the basis of negligence law.

NEGLIGENCE CLAIMS

Clinical negligence is merely the name given to negligence that arises within healthcare practice. As in any negligence claim there are two stages, the liability stage and the quantum stage.

The liability stage relates to the fact that the claimant has to establish liability on the part of the defendant, that is, that negligence has occurred; they have to prove four elements in their claim. These elements are:

- Duty of care
- Breach of that duty
- Harm
- Causation

To put it another way, the claimant, who will be a patient or their representative, has to prove that the defendant, a healthcare practitioner, owed them a duty of care; that this duty was breached because the care they received was below the necessary standard; that they suffered harm and that the harm they suffered was as a result of the low standard of care they received.

All of the above elements must be proved; if the claimant is unable to prove one of these elements, their case will fail, and no negligence will be found.

Healthcare practitioners have a duty of care to their patients. Therefore, in a claim in clinical negligence, it is generally not a difficulty for the claimant to prove that the defendant owed them a duty of care.

For a claimant to establish that the healthcare practitioner has breached their duty of care, they will have to prove that care and treatment provided by the healthcare practitioner to the patient fell below the required standard.

The required standard is often referred to as the standard of care and encompasses the professional standard as discussed in **Why is the professional standard important to a healthcare practitioner?** It also has two other elements to it. The first is to consider the defendant healthcare practitioner's practice against what other healthcare practitioners would do in the same circumstances and the second is to determine if the defendant healthcare practitioner's practice has a logical basis to it.

Both of these additional elements arise from legal cases that considered clinical negligence. Comparing the defendant healthcare practitioner's practice against other healthcare practitioners is known as the 'Bolam test' after the Bolam v Friern Hospital Management Committee [1957] case. Determining if the defendant healthcare practitioner's practice has a logical basis to it is known as the 'Bolitho test' after the Bolitho v City and Hackney Health Authority [1998] case.

A defendant healthcare practitioner's practice will meet the 'Bolam test' if other healthcare practitioners would do the same or similar in the same set of circumstances. They will meet the 'Bolitho test' if their practice can be shown to withstand logical scrutiny; this usually means that it has been based on an evidence-based approach (see **What is evidence-based practice?**), and the defendant healthcare practitioner can justify the evidence they used to inform their decision-making.

There are various types of harm that a claimant can claim for as a result of the negligent act of another including:

- Personal injury
- Damage to their property
- Monetary loss, but only as a result of one of the first two types of harm

The fact that the patient (claimant) has shown that the healthcare practitioner (defendant) owed them a duty of care, that this duty to them was breached because the healthcare practitioner's care fell below the required standard, and the patient suffered harm is not enough to successfully bring a clinical negligence claim.

Causation must also be proved, that is, that the harm suffered was directly caused by the healthcare practitioner's breach of their duty of care.

The test for proving causation is generally the 'but for' test. This test asks 'but for' the breach of duty by the healthcare practitioner, would the harm suffered by the patient have occurred? If the answer is yes, this means another factor could have caused the harm, and the patient will not be able to prove their case and will have lost their claim against the healthcare practitioner. On the other hand, if the answer is no, 'but for' the breach of duty by the healthcare practitioner the harm would not have occurred, the claimant will have proved the four elements needed, established the liability of the healthcare practitioner and won their case.

The quantum stage of a negligence case only occurs once the claimant has established the liability stage. Quantum refers to the amount of damages, the monetary award, which the defendant will have to pay to the claimant. There are various factors that are taken into account when deciding upon the damages that the claimant will receive. This includes previous cases and the damages awarded in them; however, it will be the facts of the specific case that play the major part of the calculation of damages. Damages are also known as compensation.

GROSS NEGLIGENCE MANSLAUGHTER

This is a specific criminal offence where the harm caused to the patient by the healthcare practitioner's breach of their duty of care is so severe that the patient dies. It will be tried in the criminal courts and can also result in civil action by the patient's family.

END NOTE

The vast majority of clinical negligence claims never reach court. It has been estimated that less than one in twenty are heard in court. The rest are settled out of court, with the vast majority of claims being abandoned once the healthcare practitioner has given their perspective and the health records have been checked, which highlights the importance of keeping good records (see **Is it important for healthcare practitioners to record their decisions?**)

Q Are there any special considerations in the duty of care or standard of care?

A Clinical negligence as outlined in **What is clinical negligence?** is relatively straightforward. The patient who sues a healthcare practitioner has to prove four elements or lose their case.

There are two areas which may pose an issue for healthcare practitioners, and these are in relation to the duty of care and the standard of care.

DUTY OF CARE

It is well established that healthcare practitioners owe their patients a duty of care. Also, that this duty is extended to all the patients under the care of their employer. The issue that may arise is when a healthcare practitioner feels compelled to act outside of their work environment.

One situation is acting as a Good Samaritan in an emergency in the non-work environment, for instance, the healthcare practitioner witnessing a car collision on the way home from work. There is no legal requirement for anyone to act in this kind of situation unless they already have a duty of care to the person involved. It is unlikely that the healthcare practitioner will have a duty of care to a stranger. However, although there is no legal requirement to do so, the healthcare practitioner may choose to act or realise that they are required to act by their statutory regulatory body.

Not all of the statutory regulatory bodies have this requirement but some, such as the General Medical Council and the Nursing and Midwifery Council, do. The Nursing and Midwifery Council's (2018) code states that registrants must *always offer help if an emergency arises in your practice setting or anywhere else* (at paragraph 15). This is a clear requirement that the registrant must act. Failure to act could be seen as failing to maintain the professional standard. The requirement is limited in that paragraph 15.1 requires registrants to *only act in an emergency within the limits of your knowledge and competence* while paragraph 15.3 allows the registrant to *take account of your own safety, the safety of others and the availability of other options for providing care*.

This is an issue because where a person, whether that is a healthcare practitioner or not, assumes a duty voluntarily, they assume all the potential liabilities that go along with that duty. This means that any care they give would have to meet the standard of care.

There are two positives to this assumption of the duty of care from a professional accountability perspective. The first is that the standard of care will be that of someone assisting in an emergency rather than someone who is skilled at emergency work. The second is that the government introduced the Social Action, Responsibility and Heroism Act 2015. This Act can limit a healthcare practitioner's assumed duty of care if a clinical negligence claim was brought against them for assisting in an emergency. The Act requires any court to give consideration to why the healthcare practitioner was involved and, where the reason is considered to be one that is in the public interest, to ask if it is also in the public interest to allow the duty of care to be imposed on the healthcare practitioner. If the court finds that it is not in the public interest to impose the duty, then not having a duty to a potential claimant means that the claim for clinical negligence cannot proceed; no duty of care, no clinical negligence.

STANDARD OF CARE

When discussing **What is clinical negligence?**, the standard of care was described as consisting of meeting the Bolam test and the Bolitho test. There are several types of practitioners for whom this could be problematic. These are trainees and inexperienced healthcare practitioners and those have advanced their practice beyond that normally undertaken by their professional group.

Neither the Bolam nor the Bolitho test is unchanged for these groups of healthcare practitioners but there is a change to the way that the Bolam test is applied. The Bolitho test will therefore not be considered any further in this answer.

The Bolam test requires that the practice of a healthcare practitioner is compared to other healthcare practitioners to see what they would do in the same circumstance and, only if they would do the same, has the healthcare practitioner passed the Bolam test and met the standard of care.

The question is, is it fair to judge trainee and inexperienced healthcare practitioner against the actions of other healthcare practitioner? The answer is it depends upon who those other healthcare practitioners are. Where trainee or inexperienced healthcare practitioner is being judged by the Bolam test, they are not being judged against experienced and qualified healthcare practitioners but against their peers, that is, other trainee or inexperienced healthcare practitioners. In this way, the Bolam test is a fair test.

It is only where a trainee or inexperienced healthcare practitioner is undertaking tasks outside of their expected competence that they would be judged against those healthcare practitioners who are competent to undertake that task.

This brings us to those healthcare practitioners who extend their practice beyond what is normally expected for their professional group. An example may help. Imagine Amelia and Jack are working on Fielden ward. Both are nurses, but Amelia has undergone additional education and skills training and can perform tasks and roles that Jack cannot. If Amelia were required to prove that she has met the standard of care, in assessing her using the Bolam test, she would not be compared to Jack, another nurse, but to a healthcare practitioner of the profession that normally performs that task. For instance, if Amelia were performing surgical procedures that were usually undertaken by a doctor, she would be assessed against doctors and what they would do in similar circumstances.

The implication for those healthcare practitioners who extend their practice is their peer group for assessing the Bolam test changes as their role changes. A healthcare practitioner will always be judged against healthcare practitioners who normally perform the role or task in question.

Q What is a fitness to practise investigation?

A A fitness to practise investigation is an investigation conducted by one of the statutory regulatory bodies into one of its registrants to determine if the registrant is fit, or competent, to practise. It is part of the statutory regulatory body's role in protecting the public from unfit and/or incompetent healthcare practitioners.

Statutory regulatory bodies may only initiate an investigation into possible impairment of a healthcare practitioner's fitness to practise when a concern has been raised with them or they have otherwise come into information that would raise a concern. Concerns can be raised by members of the public, patients, and former patients, colleagues of the healthcare practitioner, the healthcare practitioner's employer and other organisations including the police.

Issues that may lead to a concern include:

- A criminal conviction
- Fraudulent information or documentation
- Lack of competence
- Lack of an indemnity arrangement
- Misconduct
- Physical or mental health issues

A fitness to practise investigation has to follow a set of very detailed procedures which seek to ensure that the healthcare practitioner receives a fair and just hearing. The purpose of the fitness to practise investigation is to identify the nature of the concern that has been raised to see that it a concern they can investigate; to obtain all the relevant information, including from the healthcare practitioner; and to establish if, based on the available evidence, the concern is justified and points to a risk to public safety and/or incompetence and/or a breach of the professional standard and/or negatively affects the profession's reputation.

If the investigation determines that there is a case to answer, the case is passed to a fitness to practise hearing panel.

The fitness to practise hearing determines if the healthcare practitioner has breached the professional standard or is otherwise unfit to practise. The fitness to practise hearing is similar to a civil law case, follows set procedures and is judged on the balance of probabilities, that is, which side's argument is believed more than the others. They are generally public hearings. Healthcare practitioners can be represented in the hearing and there may be witnesses and evidence presented which the healthcare practitioner will have a right to challenge and defend.

If, as a result of a fitness to practise hearing, the healthcare practitioner is found to be unfit to practise by the tribunal, they will apply a sanction on the healthcare practitioner; see **What sanctions can be imposed by a statutory regulatory body?** for a discussion of the available sanctions. The fitness to practise hearing panel has to give reasons for their decision and for the sanction they impose.

The outcome of a fitness to practise hearing can be appealed by the healthcare practitioner against a finding of fact or against the severity of the sanction applied. The Professional Standards Authority, which oversees the statutory regulatory bodies, can appeal if they believe that the decision should not have been reached or that the fitness to practise hearing panel has been too lenient.

Q Can a healthcare practitioner be investigated for personal as well as professional issues?

A Most cases that are heard by fitness to practise committees are based on the healthcare practitioner's professional conduct or their professional competence. However, the professional standard is set in their respective codes of conduct by the statutory regulatory bodies. Anything that is covered by code of conduct that governs the healthcare practitioner can be considered by a fitness to practise investigation.

Using the term 'professional conduct', as was done in Chapter 3 in **What constitutes professional conduct?,** is a bit of a misnomer as it implies that it is only the professional aspect of a healthcare practitioner's life that is of concern. In fact, personal aspects of a healthcare practitioner's life can be considered if it affects their profession.

Some healthcare practitioners may be surprised to hear that their personal lives are covered by the code of conduct issued by their statutory regulatory body. This is because the codes of conduct have 'catch all' clauses that require the healthcare practitioner to consider how their actions affect their profession and its reputation, at all times.

The Health and Care Professions Council's (2016) code of conduct is quite explicit as under '*your duties as a registrant*' it states '*you must keep high standards of personal conduct*' while the catch-all clause is '*you must behave with honesty and integrity and make sure that your behaviour does not damage the public's confidence in you or your profession*' (at page 3).

Nursing and Midwifery Council's (2018) code states that registrants must '*uphold the reputation of your profession at all times*' (at paragraph 20).

Much as one may want to, there is no real arguing that these clauses do not cover a healthcare practitioner's conduct in their personal as well as professional lives.

Q What sanctions can be imposed by a statutory regulatory body?

A Seeing how you could be sanctioned by your statutory regulatory body is probably the last thing you want to think about. However, in brief, all of the statutory regulatory bodies have similar sanctions available to them but seem to use different language and terms to mean the same thing.

In decreasing order of severity, the available sanctions are:

- Removal of the healthcare practitioner from the professional register – commonly known as a striking off order, and the healthcare practitioner is unable to practise as a registered healthcare practitioner in that profession.
- Suspension of the healthcare practitioner from the professional register for periods of up to 12 months – generally known as a suspension order. During the

period of suspension, the healthcare practitioner is not allowed to practise as a registered healthcare practitioner in that profession.

- Placing conditions on the healthcare practitioner's practice known as a conditions of practice order. These can last for period of up to three years. The conditions that can be placed on a healthcare practitioner's practice include that they do not work within certain clinical specialties or areas; that they have to work supervised; that they do not work with certain patient groups; that they have to comply with a specified medical condition such as taking medication; that they comply with blood and/or urine drug or alcohol testing; that they undertake retraining on specified procedures or on more general aspects of practice such as dealing with difficult patients, the need for consent or how to maintain confidentiality.
- Issuing warnings and reprimands. In many ways, these are seen as lesser sanctions as they do not impinge on the healthcare practitioner's practice but let the healthcare practitioner know that their practice has not met the professional standard and, if this were to continue, they could be subject to a higher level of sanction.

Q **What should you do if, despite all your professional efforts, something does go wrong in your practice?**

A Chapter 7 examined the possible consequences of poor practice for the healthcare practitioner, and the options and processes available to patients when things go wrong in healthcare. This final thought is not about that but about you and what you should do if you are involved in an adverse event.

Hopefully by now, assuming you haven't just jumped straight to this question, you will be able to answer this question yourself and you are only asking it to confirm what you already know.

So what should you do if something goes wrong? The big thing to remember is communication.

You need to inform people, many people, and as soon as you can after ensuring the patient is as safe as they can be.

Initially your priority should be your patient and their safety and getting whatever assistance you need.

Who should you be communicating with: fellow healthcare practitioners in your team, your line manager, your supervisor/mentor, your employer and/or your university department. You need to let people know what has happened so that any appropriate steps can be taken to rectify the issues.

You may also want to communicate with the patient to let them know what has happened, what will be happening to put it right and to say sorry if appropriate.

Once the immediate aftermath of the event has been dealt with, you may need to communicate with your employer's legal department, your union and/or your indemnity provider. At this stage, your priority is ensuring that you receive appropriate advice and guidance.

Later on, you will need to communicate with any other healthcare practitioners involved in the event and reflect upon what happened, what may have caused the event, your part in the event and how you can learn from it and what you may do differently in the future. You may need to share these reflections with others as part of a formal investigation or for the purposes of wider quality assurance and risk management.

Your reflection should allow you to have a plan as what you would do the same and what you would do differently if the same set of circumstances were to recur in the future.

But remember, the more prepared you are for your practice, the more professional you are in your approach to practice and your patients, the less likely that an adverse event will occur. Also, there are many sources of support for you, and you should avail yourself of these. There is no reason to face any of the possible consequences of poor practice or a mistake or an adverse event on your own.

SUMMARY

- There are various ways in which a healthcare practitioner may be involved if something goes wrong in healthcare. These include complaints, civil and criminal legal cases, employer disciplinary proceedings and fitness to practise investigations.
- Healthcare practitioners have a duty under their professional accountability to challenge poor practice.
- Raising a concern is not always easy but there are sources of support and guidance for healthcare practitioners.
- Whistleblowing is a very specific means of raising a concern. There are legal protections for healthcare practitioners who follow the necessary conditions.
- While mistakes are not wanted, they can provide learning experiences for healthcare practitioners.
- The duty of candour exists to instil a culture of openness, honesty and transparency into healthcare, especially when things go wrong.
- The statutory duty of candour only applies to healthcare organisations. The professional duty of candour applies to healthcare practitioners and is a requirement of the statutory regulatory bodies.
- It is part of a healthcare practitioner's professional accountability to say sorry to a patient when a mistake happens. Doing so does not impose a liability where none previously existed.
- Complaints are a part of the quality assurance in healthcare. If a healthcare practitioner receives a complaint, they should ensure they follow their local policy in responding to it.
- Healthcare practitioners may be required to provide statements to a Coroner's Court, whose function is to determine who died and when, where and how the death occurred.

- Clinical negligence is when a patient sues a healthcare practitioner because they have breached their duty of care to the patient by giving them care that is below the required standard, and the patient has suffered harm as a result of this substandard care.
- If a healthcare practitioner acts outside of their work environment, they will assume a duty of care where none previously existed.
- When healthcare practitioners are judged by the Bolam test to determine if they have met the standard of care, they will always be judged against the professional group who normally performs the role or task in question.
- Fitness to practise investigations determine if a healthcare practitioner has breached their professional standard and pose a risk to the public and, if so, may lead to a fitness to practise hearing which could ultimately lead to the healthcare practitioner being sanctioned by the statutory regulatory body.
- Because of a requirement by the statutory regulatory body's codes of conduct to always uphold their profession's reputation, healthcare practitioners can be investigated for personal as well as professional issues.
- The statutory regulatory bodies have a range of sanctions available to them, ranging from warnings to removal of the healthcare practitioner from the professional register.
- If something does go wrong within your practice, remember to ensure that you communicate with relevant individuals, including the patient, to ensure that the patient is safe and receives the appropriate assistance, and that you receive appropriate advice and guidance.

REFERENCES

Bolam v Friern Hospital Management Committee [1957] 2 All ER 118.

Bolitho v City and Hackney Health Authority [1998] AC 232.

Campbell, D. (2013) 'Mid staffs hospital scandal: The essential guide', *The Guardian*. Available at: https://www.theguardian.com/society/2013/feb/06/mid-staffs-hospital-scandal-guide

Chief Executives of Statutory Regulators of Healthcare Professionals (2014) *Openness and Honesty – The Professional Duty of Candour*. Available at: https://www.gcc-uk.org/assets/publications/Joint_statement_on_the_professional_duty_of_candour.pdf

Compensation Act 2006.

Coroners Act 1988.

Coroners Rules 1984.

Department of Health (2000) *An Organisation with a Memory*. Department of Health: London.

Department of Health (2014) *Hard Truths: The Journey to Putting Patients First* Cm-8777-I and Cm 8711-II. Department of Health: London.

Donoghue v Stevenson [1932] AC 562.

Health and Care Professions Council (2016) *Standards of Conduct, Performance and Ethics*. Health and Care Professions Council: London.

Mid Staffordshire NHS Foundation Trust Public Inquiry (2013) *Report of the Mid Staffordshire NHS foundation trust public inquiry: executive summary* (HC 947). The

Stationery Office: London. Available at: http://www.midstaffspublicinquiry.com/sites/default/files/report/Executive%20summary.pdf

Nursing and Midwifery Council (2018) *The code*. Nursing and Midwifery Council: London.

Public Interest Disclosure Act 1998.

Social Action, Responsibility and Heroism Act 2015.

The Health and Social Care Act 2008 (Regulated Activities) Regulations 2014 (SI 2014/2936).

A FINAL QUESTION

Q So overall, what does it mean to be an accountable healthcare professional?

A An accountable healthcare professional is one who:

- Is aware that they are in a position of privilege and trust
- Adopts the values of their profession
- Practises according to the professional standard
- Is professionally accountable
- Is registered with one of the statutory regulatory bodies
- Maintains their clinical competence and does not practise outside of their competence
- Undertakes continuing professional development and revalidation as required
- Works as part of a healthcare team in a collaborative manner
- Respects the rights of their patients and advocates for them as necessary
- Adopts a shared decision-making approach
- Utilises evidence in their decision-making
- Raises concerns about colleagues and resources when necessary
- Challenges poor practice
- Knows what to do if something goes wrong
- Is open honest and transparent with patients if mistakes occur
- Uses mistakes and complaints as a learning opportunity